Small Animal Radiographic Techniques and Positioning

Small Animal Radiographic Techniques and Positioning

Mary H. (Susie) Ayers BBA, RT(R)

Illustrations by L. Ashley Marlowe

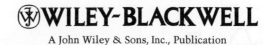

A John Wiley & Sons, Inc., Publication

This edition first published 2012 © 2012 by John Wiley & Sons, Inc.

Wiley-Blackwell is an imprint of John Wiley & Sons, formed by the merger of Wiley's global Scientific, Technical and Medical business with Blackwell Publishing.

Registered office: John Wiley & Sons Ltd, The Atrium, Southern Gate, Chichester, West Sussex, PO19 8SQ, UK

Editorial offices: 2121 State Avenue, Ames, Iowa 50014-8300, USA
The Atrium, Southern Gate, Chichester, West Sussex, PO19 8SQ, UK
9600 Garsington Road, Oxford, OX4 2DQ, UK

For details of our global editorial offices, for customer services and for information about how to apply for permission to reuse the copyright material in this book please see our website at www.wiley.com/wiley-blackwell.

Library of Congress Cataloging-in-Publication Data

Ayers, Mary H.
    Small animal radiographic techniques and positioning / Mary H. (Susie) Ayers ; illustrations by L. Ashley Marlowe.
        p. ; cm.
    Includes bibliographical references and index.
    ISBN 978-0-8138-1152-9 (pbk. : alk. paper)
    I. Title.
    [DNLM: 1. Radiography–veterinary.   2. Animal Diseases–diagnosis.   3. Diagnostic Imaging–methods.   4. Patient Positioning–veterinary.   5. Technology, Radiologic–veterinary.   SF 757.8]
    632'.9–dc23
                            2011035810

A catalogue record for this book is available from the British Library.

Set in 10/12 pt Sabon by Toppan Best-set Premedia Limited

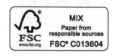

To my husband, Gene,
for all of his love and support, today and every day.

Contents

> **Companion website**
> This book is accompanied by a companion website:
> www.wiley.com/go/ayers

Foreword

Susie Ayers has been teaching veterinary students the science and art of veterinary radiography for many, many years. She has witnessed a remarkable evolution in how veterinarians and veterinary technicians practice our profession, especially in the imaging sciences. Her experiences and, perhaps more importantly, her passion for her career have brought us an enjoyably readable handbook, *Small Animal Radiographic Techniques and Positioning*. It blends the new with the old, provides helpful tips and words of caution, supported with color photography, illustrative line drawings, and excellent quality radiographic images. Students especially will embrace the friendly, non-"textbook" style and find the "how-to" special procedures section very useful in practice.

John S. Mattoon, DVM, Dipl ACVR
Professor and Chief of Radiology
Department of Veterinary Clinical Sciences
Washington State University
Pullman, Washington

Preface

It has been such a privilege to work in veterinary imaging for 23 years with veterinary students and veterinary technicians. The veterinary technician's role has grown as technology and advancements in medicine have progressed over the years. Today, the veterinary technician scope of practice includes not only nursing care but also anesthesia, laboratory, and diagnostic imaging responsibilities. Small animal practices are growing and purchasing more advanced imaging equipment and their techs are expected to expand their roles to become proficient in operating the equipment. When veterinary technicians graduate and enter the workplace, they may work in a practice still manually processing film or be expected to know how to operate digital imaging equipment. This handbook is written for both the veterinary technician and the small animal practitioner to assist them with the varied imaging challenges they may encounter in today's working environment.

The book is divided into three sections, covering an overview of radiographic technique, darkroom maintenance, digital and film-screen imaging in the first section; small animal positioning, including some exotic species positioning techniques, in the second section; and contrast media and special contrast enhanced procedures in the last section. The intent of the text is to provide a one-stop handbook to quickly find needed imaging information, whether it is the correct contrast media dose for a special procedure or a quick lookup for positioning.

Acknowledgments

I would like to acknowledge some very special people at the Virginia-Maryland Regional College of Veterinary Medicine and Veterinary Teaching Hospital at Virginia Tech for their support and contributions over the past year. Many thanks go to my friend Carolyn Sink, who suggested I should write this text. I would also like to thank Dr. F. William Pierson, the VTH Hospital Director, for access to our digital image files. I also appreciate the advice, suggestions, and support given by our radiologists, Dr. Gregory Daniel, Dr. Martha Larson, and Dr. Reid Tyson. Special thanks to Dr. Reid Tyson and his family pet, Kona, for the alternative restraint demonstration pictures. I would also like to thank three other special radiologists for their contributions, Dr. Donald L. Barber, Dr. Jeryl Jones, and Dr. Colin Carrig. Also, I appreciate the imaging cases contributed by department staff technologists Valerie and Becki.

I want to especially thank Dr. Richard Bryant, owner of Salem Animal Hospital and VT alumni, for generously allowing me access to his practice to take darkroom and radiographic room pictures. I would like to thank my illustrator, Ashley Marlowe, for doing such a terrific job on this project. She juggled her studies while doing my illustrations, using her dog, Charley, as her model. I am truly blessed to have met her years ago in church and have watched her grow to become such a talented artist. I would also like to thank my sister, Erma Chambers, for her assistance and advice in helping me navigate the publishing unknowns. Another very important person to acknowledge is my husband, Gene. He has continuously provided encouragement and support throughout the process.

Lastly, I cannot leave out my pets, feathered and furry, for their contributions to this book. Some of them were adopted from the vet school and have been cared for by some terrific clinicians, senior veterinary students, and veterinary technicians while being patients at the VTH. They have never complained when taken to work with me to allow students to practice handling and imaging. Special thanks to Valerie's Reuben, who unknowingly contributed some great images for the text. Also, I must acknowledge my beloved pet and companion of 13 years, Charley, who passed away in 2011. His image file provided material for the text and he faithfully sat next to me while I was writing. You will always be in my heart.

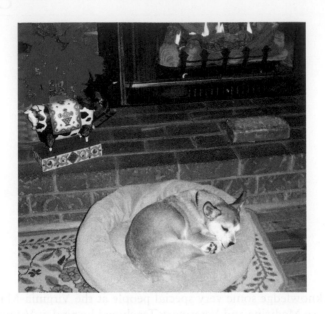

Small Animal
Radiographic Techniques
and Positioning

Section 1

Theory and Equipment

Introduction to Digital Imaging

Small animal radiography has changed dramatically in the past decade with the appearance of digital radiography in veterinary medicine. Many small animal practices that were hand developing x-ray film have taken the next step to automatic x-ray film processing due to the availability of affordable used and new tabletop x-ray film processors and faster x-ray film-screen cassette combinations. Switching to 400 speed rare earth film-screen combinations has decreased radiation exposure to technical staff and the patient, as well as improved the quality of the images due to shorter x-ray exposure times.

As digital radiography (**DR**) has become more affordable, an increasing number of small animal practices have switched from film-screen imaging to digital radiography. The list of vendors marketing veterinary digital radiographic systems is growing, so a variety of options are available from an economic perspective. Some vendors have products utilizing older digital technology; therefore it is important for small animal practitioners and their technical staff to have a basic understanding of digital radiography to assist in choosing the right digital radiographic system for their practices and also to have the needed knowledge to improve the quality of the digital radiographic images being taken.[6]

Definition and Principles of Digital Imaging

Digital imaging is simply an imaging acquisition process that generates an electronic image to be viewed and manipulated on a computer. All types of medical images are produced in a digital format including computed tomography (**CT**), ultrasound, magnetic resonance imaging (**MRI**), nuclear medicine, digital fluoroscopy, computed radiography (**CR**), and digital radiography direct and indirect capture.[4,5]

Digital Radiography

Digital radiography is a term used to reference the two main systems used in both human and veterinary medicine, computed radiography and digital (direct capture or indirect capture) radiography.[1,4,5] Digital radiography is constantly changing as improvements to this technology are being made through both software and hardware.

Digital Imaging Communications in Medicine

Digital imaging communications in medicine (**DICOM**) is the image file format that standardizes medical digital images from all imaging modalities and picture archiving and communication systems from different manufacturers. If different vendors used proprietary formats, images could not be sent to other facilities using different software to view the images. When purchasing a digital radiographic system, it is important to make sure the system comes with a DICOM conformance statement.[1,5,8] A DICOM conformance statement describes exactly how the software or device conforms to the DICOM standard. The statement follows a standard format to allow a user or vendor to determine if two devices will communicate and are compatible by comparing conformance statements.

Picture Archiving and Communication System

A picture archiving and communication system (**PACS**) provides image capture, display, annotation, archival, and communication functions allowing the images to be viewed at multiple computer workstations in a practice. Long-term storage of digital images is important because the data is part of the patient's medical record. Veterinary practices can purchase affordable small PACS to permit viewing in exams rooms and surgery. Since the image format is DICOM, there will be no problem sending the images to another practitioner or a referral facility.

There is a rather wide selection of storage device options to choose from, each differing in data access, storage capacity, and cost for both onsite and off-site storage.[7] For onsite storage, some practices just choose to use hard disk drives with a backup and invest in a web-based PACS service. Using a web-based PACS provides the small animal practitioner with the capability to permit a referral practice to view the DICOM images taken on a patient from anywhere in the world. An email can be sent to the specialty veterinary practice with the link to download the DICOM images for review, thereby allowing the specialist quick access to DICOM images. It should be noted it may take up to 24 hours before images are available for viewing on some web-based PACS services. This isn't a common problem in recent years, but it is an important question to ask when planning to purchase a contract with a web-based PACS service. Emailing images is not recommended if it is necessary to convert the DICOM image to a jpeg or tiff due to loss of detail in the image. Sending DICOM images via CD or DVD is the secondary preferred method when it is necessary to send images to a specialty practice that is not set up to accept emailed DICOM links.

Workstation Monitors

To adequately review images taken, it has been recommended to have a medical grade grayscale monitor as part of the primary display workstation, particularly in a specialty practice. This thought has been changing over the past 5 years because the newer high-end consumer grade color monitors are just as bright as their medical grade counterparts and they also have an acceptable resolution. At the 2006 Radiological Society of North America (**RSNA**) conference, Dr. David Hirshorn MD stated in a presentation that the differences in interpretation between a properly calibrated high-end consumer grade display and a medical grade grayscale display were not statistically significant.[19] Top-quality color monitors are brighter than the normal grade consumer monitor and have a brightness greater than 400–500 cd/m^2 and a contrast ratio of at least 800:1–1000:1.[19] The advantage of the medical grade grayscale monitor over the consumer grade high-quality display monitor is greater monitor stability. Thus a consumer grade monitor may be sufficient for the basic small animal practice. The choice depends upon the type of practice and the financial investment the practice can afford.

For a practitioner to visualize a digital image of similar quality to a film image necessitates the display monitor to have high spatial resolution (recorded detail).[3] For the primary display workstation utilizing a medical grade monitor, the small animal practitioner should ideally use a 2K (2MP) resolution portrait monitor. The common screen resolutions for medical display monitors are 1280 × 1024 (1K/1MP), 1600 × 1200 (2K/2MP), 2048 × 1536 (3K/3MP), and 2048 × 2560 (5K/5MP).[1,3] CR and DR images are generally best viewed on at least a 2K/2MP monitor, whereas cross-sectional images can be viewed on a 1K/1MP monitor. Radiologists generally use at least a 3K/3MP or above for reading digital images. Viewing on a 3MP monitor eliminates the need to zoom or pan the images to review all of the details in the image (Figs. 1.1a and 1.1b).

There are some basic terms that need to be defined to allow a better understanding of how these monitors work. A basic picture element is called a **pixel**. Each pixel is a set of **dot triads**. A dot triad is a grouping of one red dot, one green dot, and one blue dot. **Bit depth** is used to describe the number of bits used to store information about each pixel of

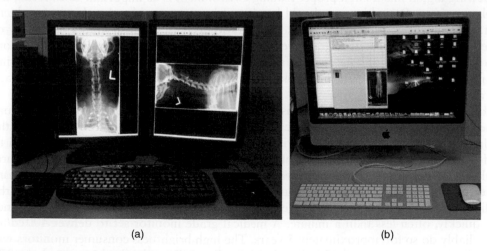

(a)   (b)

Figure 1.1   a. DR workstation with medical grade monitors. b. Mac workstation.

an image.[19] The bit depth of an image will determine how many levels of gray or color can be generated. For example, a digital camera generally has 24- to 32-bit color. Digital radiographic systems have only 10–16 bits of grayscale. So a 24-bit color system will have one-third of that for each color or 8 bits (256 shades) of each color that can be combined to produce millions of colors. To produce a shade of gray the intensity of each of the three colors must be exactly equal, which means a 24-bit color camera can only produce 256 shades (8 bits) of gray.[19] Pixels are arranged in a **matrix,** a rectangular or square table of numbers that represents the pixel intensity to be displayed on the monitor.[1] Examples are 2048 × 1536 and 2048 × 2560, the most common matrices for image viewing by a veterinary radiologist. **Dot pitch** is the measurement of how close the dots are located to one another within a pixel. The number of pixels on a monitor's display is known as its **resolution.** As the dot pitch of a display becomes smaller, resolution improves.[1] The greater the number of pixels in an image, the higher the resolution, which means more information can be displayed. Brightness or luminance refers to how bright the image appears on a display.[19] The brighter the display, the greater dynamic range produced in the image. A greater dynamic range will allow you to resolve more shades of gray in the image and is necessary to provide a full 8-bit grayscale image or 256 distinct shades of gray. If the maximum brightness of a display is inadequate, adjacent shades of gray will not be distinguishable and subtle lesions may be missed. A monitor used for primary diagnosis should be at least 400–500 cd/m^2 brightness.[19] **Contrast ratio** describes the difference between the blacks and the whites that a monitor can display. Any monitor used for primary diagnosis should have a contrast ratio of at least 1000:1, which means the black on the display is 1,000 times darker than the white on the display.[19] Another important measurement to use in choosing a monitor is its **refresh rate.** The refresh rate is the number of times an image is rewritten on the monitor each second. The refresh rate controls the flicker seen by the viewer so a high refresh rate is preferable when selecting a monitor. The most common refresh rates set on computer monitors are between 60 and 75 Hz, which means the image is refreshed 60–75 times per second. When searching for a monitor, **aspect ratio** and **viewable area** are two other terms you need to know. The aspect ratio is simply the ratio of the width to the height of the monitor. The viewable area of a monitor is determined by measuring the front of the display diagonally from one corner to the other.[1]

Viewing digital images in a proper reading environment is as important as choosing the display monitor. Digital images should be viewed in a room with a low level of ambient light. As ambient light increases, the contrast ratio decreases, which means the ability of the eye to distinguish between gray levels is best when the ambient light level of the room is close to the amount of light coming from the screen. Also, the viewer should be viewing the monitor at eye level and not looking down or up at the monitor to avoid image degradation.[19]

Monitor stability should also be considered when choosing whether to purchase a consumer grade color monitor or a medical grade grayscale display monitor. Stabilizing the luminance of the backlight(s) is essential in the monitor's ability to be calibrated and to hold the calibration. The LCD backlight will vary in luminance over time and temperature. It takes time for an LCD monitor to warm up and stabilize after being turned on. A consumer grade monitor can take over an hour to reach maximum luminance versus the medical grade monitor, which is designed to bring the backlight to its calibrated luminance very quickly, often less than a minute. A medical grade monitor set to deliver 400 cd/m^2 will reliably do so for approximately 5 years. The high brightness consumer monitors will generally have an output of 450 cd/m^2, initially, but will gradually decay to about 375 cd/m^2 in about 18 months.[19] What does this mean? The consumer grade monitor, due to its lack of stability, will only be diagnostically useful for about a third of the time of a medical grade display. But the consumer grade monitor only costs a fraction of the cost of a medical grade monitor. So if a high-quality consumer grade color display will suit the needs of the practice, it may be the best choice from an economic perspective, understanding the monitor will need to be replaced on a more frequent basis.

Regardless of the display chosen, the monitor must be regularly calibrated. It is necessary to do so because LCD monitors degrade over time. The LCD screen is illuminated by a backlight that is constantly on at full intensity. As stated earlier, the luminance of this backlight will decrease over time, due to the phosphors in the lamp wearing out. Some monitor vendors may supply test patterns, software, and sensors to perform visual tests. External hardware and sensors can also be purchased. Information for the practitioner regarding medical display acceptance testing and quality control can be found on the American Association of Physicists in Medicine (**AAPM**), Task Group 18's website, http:// deckard.mc.duke.edu/~samei/tg18. Task Group 18 consists of medical imaging experts and organizational affiliates who produced the document *Assessment of Display Performance for Medical Imaging Systems*. An excellent quick resource for information regarding DR systems for veterinary medicine, including monitor calibration, can also be found at www.animalinsides.com/htm.[19]

Cathode ray tube (**CRT**) and liquid crystal display (**LCD**) are the most common types of monitors currently used in a medical setting, though plasma monitors are increasing in popularity. LCD and plasma monitors should be familiar because most of the TVs on the market today are either LCD or plasma.

CRT monitors have a cathode and an anode located within a vacuum tube that works in a similar fashion to an x-ray tube. The advantages of the CRT monitor are they are less expensive, more durable than the LCD or plasma monitors, and have better color representation and superior resolution. The aspect ratio of a CRT monitor is 4:3. The disadvantages of the CRT monitors are they take up a lot of space, are heavy, are not easily adjustable for viewing at different heights and angles, and emit heat.[1]

LCD monitors are used more and more as they have decreased in cost and increased in quality in recent years. The advantages of the LCD monitor arc they take up less space, use less power than a CRT monitor, are lighter weight, produce less heat, and the surface produces little glare. The aspect ratio of an LCD monitor is 16:9. The disadvantages are they cost more than a CRT monitor and have less of a viewing angle, the display is not as bright as the CRT, and each display is only capable of working with a single physical resolution.

Plasma displays contain many small fluorescent lights that are illuminated to form the color of the image. The plasma display varies the intensities of the various light combinations to produce a full range of color. The advantages are they require a smaller frame around the display, have a wide screen with thin depth, are brighter than the LCD, can be viewed at varying angles, and are light weight. The disadvantages are the high cost and low availability.[1]

Of the three monitors, LCD monitors are used more in the PACS display market due to their size, resolution, and lack of heat production. The workstation receives images from the archive and/or from the digital radiographic system. The workstation has PACS application software that allows the practitioner to view and manipulate the image. It would depend upon the type of small animal practice, caseload, and specialty to determine if more than one primary display workstation would be needed. One primary workstation with either a 24 inch, 2K/2MP medical grade grayscale monitor or a high-quality consumer grade color monitor with a brightness of at least 450 cd/m^2 with a contrast ratio of 1,000:1 placed in a low-level ambient lit viewing area of the practice may suffice the needs of the practice. Monitors used for secondary viewing in surgery or in the exam room, after the diagnosis has been made, can be consumer grade 19 or 21 inch LCD panels of lesser quality than the primary. The larger dual panels may be helpful for surgery.[19]

Computed Radiography

Computed radiography was first introduced in the early 1980s by Fuji Medical Systems. CR is a cassette-based system containing an imaging plate instead of the conventional film-screen combination. Some advantages of CR are the cassette can be used in a similar fashion to the conventional x-ray film cassette and no major alteration to the existing x-ray system is required. The CR cassette can be placed on either the tabletop or in the cassette Bucky with a grid. When used tabletop, lead strips or strict collimation can allow two separate exposures to be made on the same cassette prior to processing. Whereas an x-ray film cassette is taken to a darkroom, the film is removed, stamped with the patient's name, and then sent through an x-ray film processor, the CR cassette is placed in a machine called a reader.

When the CR cassette is placed in a reader, the reader removes the imaging plate from the cassette and scans it with a red laser in a zigzag pattern called a **raster** to release the stored electrons. As the plate travels through the reader, the laser scans across the imaging plate multiple times in a process called **translation**. This scanning process produces lines of light intensity information that are detected by a photomultiplier/charge-coupled device (**CCD**) that connects the light to an electronic signal. The signal is digitized by an analog-to-digital converter (**ADC**). The ADC assigns each picture element or pixel a numerical value that corresponds to its level of brightness and position. The entire image is divided into a matrix of pixels based on the brightness of each pixel. As the number of pixels in a matrix increases for the same field of view, the smaller the pixels have to fit into the area. The smaller the pixels are in size the greater the spatial resolution.[1,3]

Spatial resolution is defined as the amount of detail in any image. Just as the crystal size and thickness of the phosphor layer determine the resolution in film-screen radiography, the phosphor layer and pixel size determine the resolution in a CR image. The thinner the phosphor layer, the higher the resolution. The unit of measuring spatial resolution is line pairs per millimeter (**lp/mm**). An x-ray test pattern, which consists of a series of lead strips separated by equal-size interspaces, is imaged. The higher the number of line pairs visualized, the greater the spatial resolution, and the smaller the detail that can be detected in an image. Film-screen images have excellent spatial resolution, measuring 10 lp/mm.[3] CR typically has 2.55–5 lp/mm resolution, which results in less detail than a film-screen image. The loss of spatial resolution is compensated for by the increase in **contrast resolution**, which refers to the proficiency of an imaging system to distinguish between small objects or tissues having similar tissue density, like liver and spleen. Many more densities or shades of gray are recorded in CR images, which increases the contrast resolution.[1,3]

After the reading process is complete, most of the electrons return to a lower energy state, which basically removes the image from the plate. The imaging plate still should be cleared at least every 48 hours by the CR reader erasure mode to prevent a buildup of background signal. CR plates are very sensitive to background and scatter radiation. After the CR plate has been read, the signal is sent to the computer, where it is preprocessed. The data appears on the monitor for review and is then sent to a PACS.

Direct and Indirect Conversion Radiography

Digital radiography can be a confusing term because it includes both computed and direct and indirect methods of digital image capture. The more accurate term is direct digital radiography (DDR), which is now commonly abbreviated as DR.[5] The DR panel is typically hard-wired to the image processing system and cassetteless, though very recently Carestream Health and Fuji Medical Systems have each released to market a wireless DR panel that can be used in conventional film-screen x-ray systems.

In hard-wired DR detectors, the materials used for detecting the x-ray signal and the sensors are permanently enclosed in a protective housing and referred to as a **flat-panel detector**. The flat-panel detector is comprised of a photoconductor such as amorphous selenium (a-Se), which changes the x-ray photons directly into an electronic signal. Silicon and CCD detectors are also included in this category, though they are older technology[1,4] (Fig. 1.2).

With the direct conversion process x-ray photons are absorbed by a photo-conducting material, such as a-SE, and converted to electrons, which are stored in thin-film transistor (**TFT**) detectors. The TFT detector is an array or grouping of small pixels with each pixel containing a photodiode. A **photodiode** is a photoelectric semiconductor device that absorbs the electrons and generates electrical charges.[5] A field-effect transistor (**FET**), which is a nonrectifying transistor, or silicon TFT, isolates each pixel element and works like a switch to send the electrical charges to the image processor.[1] The information is sent onto the data columns and read out with dedicated electronics. Silicon integrated circuits are connected to the edges of the detector matrix. Integrated circuits control the line scanning sequence on one side and low noise, high sensitivity amplifiers carry out the readout, amplification, and analog to digital conversion function on the opposite side.[1]

Indirect conversion detectors are comparable to direct detectors in that they use TFT detectors but dissimilar to direct conversion because they require a two-step process to convert to electrons and send to the image processor. With both direct and indirect

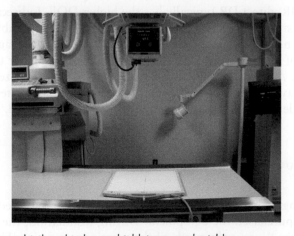

Figure 1.2.   Canon DR panel tethered to be used tabletop or under table.

conversion over one million pixels can be read and converted to a composite digital image in less than 1 second.[1]

It is recommended to avoid purchasing DR systems utilizing older technology. This older technology information is being included to assist the practitioner in identifying older systems that may still be offered by some vendors. The older indirect conversion DR system is based on CCDs. A charge-coupled device is basically a semiconductor device used as an optical sensor that stores a charge and then sequentially transfers it. In this case, the x-ray photons strike a scintillation material, such as a photostimulable phosphor or a CsI scintillator, and this signal is coupled by lenses that work like cameras. These cameras reduce the size of the projected visible light image and transfer the image to one or more small CCDs that convert the light into an electrical charge. The charge is stored in a sequential pattern and released line by line and sent to an analog-to-digital converter).[1,3]

Complementary metal oxide silicon (**CMOS**) systems use specialized pixel sensors. When these sensors are struck with x-ray photons, they convert the x-rays to light photons and store them in capacitors. Each pixel has its own amplifier, which is turned off and on by circuitry within the pixel converting the light photons into electrical charges. Voltage from the amplifier is converted by an analog-to-digital converter, also located within the pixel. The system was developed by NASA and is both extremely efficient and takes up less fill space than CCDs.[1,3]

When choosing a digital radiographic system it is important to ask about the detective quantum efficiency of the detector. **Detective quantum efficiency (DQE)** is basically how efficiently a system converts the x-ray input signal into a useful output image.[1] DQE looks at the effects of noise and contrast on the digital image. Electronic and quantum noise are always present in digital imaging. The effect of noise is usually referred to as **signal-to-noise ratio (SNR)**. A higher-quality image consists of more signal and less noise. So high SNR captures the most useful image information and provides a higher-quality image.

In DR, contrast refers to the system's ability to accurately reproduce an object's actual contrast. Digital detectors have a wide dynamic range so they can capture a large range of intensities. Their ability to produce high contrast resolution means they can display thousands of shades of gray that can be enhanced with automatic contrast enhancement and window/leveling parameters. The ultimate goal of a system is to have a high DQE, which allows the ability to image small low contrast objects.[1,3,4]

Direct and indirect DR detectors have an increased DQE over CR systems. In comparing direct and indirect DR, direct DR typically has the higher DQE. Indirect DR systems using the newer CMOS instead of CCDs in their panels are more comparable to the direct DR systems. Keep in mind the DQE of detectors changes with kilovoltage peak (**kVp**), but normally the DQE of selenium and phosphor-based systems is higher than for CR, CCD, and CMOS systems. Another factor that increases the DQE is the size of the area of the TFT photodiode array. The greater the size of the TFT array the greater the DQE because the more radiation detected increases the amount of signal generated.[1,3,4]

Digital Image Processing

The basic digital imaging principles and equipment have been reviewed and the veterinarian has chosen and purchased the equipment. During installation, the vendor will set up the computer software to meet the needs of the veterinary practice (Fig. 1.3).

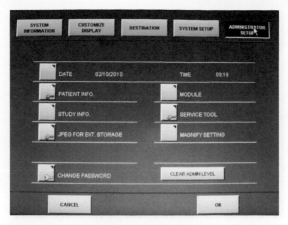

Figure 1.3. DR system administrator setup window.

The vendor will need to know which direction the patient is typically placed on the radiographic table so the orientation can be set up in the computer. This will allow the Right (R) and Left (L) anatomic notation to appear correctly on the image, if the patient is placed correctly on the table. The vendor will put the name of the practice on the image and the view taken (example: VD Thorax, Oblique Mandible, or CrCD Stifle). If the practice is a specialty practice, there may be specialized views that the vendor will need to set up in the menu or additional information to be added to each displayed image.

It is important to provide an overview of the digital imaging process once the patient is positioned on the radiographic table. Digital imaging will greatly reduce the amount of time normally needed to image a patient. For the technician, learning to use the equipment efficiently is the next step. Utilizing a DICOM modality worklist (**DICOM MWL**) will decrease the errors frequently caused by entering patient information directly into the DR system at the time the patient is to be imaged. A DICOM MWL is a bridge to the practice management software that eliminates the need for technicians to enter patient information into the DR system. If not using a DICOM worklist, it starts with entering the patient's information into the computer and selecting the correct anatomic region of interest prior to taking the exposure. It is imperative to enter complete patient identification information correctly. When a large referral practice receives images on "Charley" with no last name associated, particularly jpeg or tiff files on a CD, sent to their PACS administrator to load images onto their PACS system, it is often difficult to trace the last name, which delays the specialists' ability to view the images on their workstations. The accession number assigned to the patient when the images were taken helps the original practice to find the patient but is not helpful for the referring practice unless complete information is present. If the practice uses a DICOM modality worklist and the images are sent via an email with a DICOM link or DICOM images are sent via CD, it greatly expedites the transfer of images to the specialty practice's PACS for viewing.

Each anatomic region has a processing algorithm specific to that region for reconstructing the image prior to it being displayed on the computer screen. A processing algorithm is simply a mathematical formula that makes adjustments to the image data so the resulting image has been properly reconstructed.[1] If doing abdominal imaging, with or without using contrast media, you must choose the abdominal algorithm and not the thorax algorithm or the image data will not be properly processed (Fig. 1.4).

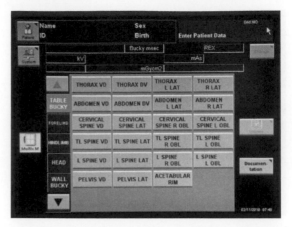

Figure 1.4.   Example of anatomic region and patient data entry page in a DR system.

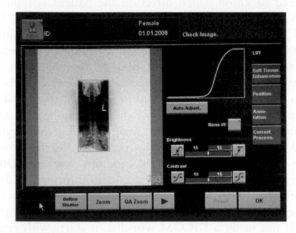

Figure 1.5.   DR image review and QA adjustment page.

Prior to the image being displayed, a histogram or graph showing the distribution of pixel values for that particular image is constructed. If the histogram indicates a high or low exposure, the image brightness will automatically be adjusted to correct the error. After the histogram evaluation, a **lookup table (LUT)** can be used to further alter the digital image to change the image density and shades of gray to manipulate how the anatomic region of interest appears. Of course this will also alter the image's brightness and contrast. The lookup table, which is a graph, will appear as a straight line if the image is not changed. If it is changed, it will have a curve similar to that of a film-screen image. This feature is mentioned because the ability to use this function is available. Please remember any change to the digital image prior to accepting the image and sending it to the primary workstation may decrease the veterinarian's ability to manipulate the image once it goes to the workstation. It is very rare that the image should be altered in any way other than possibly changing the orientation of the image on the screen before transferring it to the primary workstation (Fig. 1.5).

Another feature is changing the orientation of the image. If the image is oriented incorrectly, it will be necessary to flip or rotate the image horizontally or vertically so it appears correctly before sending the image to the primary workstation for the veterinarian to review. There will be a function menu or tab named Position or Image Orientation on the Quality Assurance (QA) page or on a toolbar that will allow the patient orientation to be changed. Also under QA, there should also be a Zoom function to allow you to review the image prior to sending. There may be a Shuttering function that will allow post-exposure collimating. If the area of interest was not collimated well using the collimator on the x-ray tube, you will have the ability to correct this to a degree on the computer. To avoid excessive backscatter radiation and to improve the quality of the image, there is NO substitution for collimating to the area of interest with the collimator on the x-ray tube, but this feature in the QA function on the computer will help. A Region of Interest (ROI) tab is generally available, also. If on the small computer screen it appears that the anatomic part is not well visualized or too dark, using the ROI function will adjust the image to a viewable brightness level. Again this tends to happen when the milliampere seconds (mAs) and kVp are too high and the histogram could not adjust appropriately. Also using the ROI function will affect what the veterinarian can adjust once the image is sent to the primary workstation for review. Using a technique chart to choose the correct technical factors and collimating to the anatomic part appropriately should prevent the necessity of using the Shutter and ROI functions. Once all the changes are complete, send the image to the primary workstation.

Principles of Film-Screen Radiography

X-ray Film Construction

Conventional film-screen radiography is still the most widely used method of imaging in small animal practices. The x-ray beam exits the x-ray tube, passes through the patient, and strikes the film-screen cassette (Fig. 2.1).

Double emulsion x-ray film is placed in a cassette containing two radiographic intensifying screens. Double emulsion radiographic film has emulsion coated on both sides of the base, and a layer of supercoat or overcoat tops off each emulsion (Fig. 2.2).

The first coat is a supercoat, overcoat, or abrasion layer, which is an outside layer protecting the emulsion from scratches, pressure, and contamination during handling, processing, and storage. The next layer is the emulsion layer, which is the radiation- and light-sensitive layer of the film. It consists of silver halide crystals suspended in gelatin. Silver halide is the material that is sensitive to radiation and light. The formulations of silver halide used by film manufacturers are proprietary but basically silver bromide (AgBr) and silver iodide (AgI) make up the emulsion layer, with approximately 90–99% constituted by silver bromide and 1–10% by silver iodide. Companies manufacturing film are using tabular grain (T-grain) technology. Instead of using randomly shaped silver halide crystals, T-grain films use flat silver halide crystals that can be more evenly dispersed in the emulsion layer gelatin to increase the recorded detail in the radiograph. The final layer is the base layer, which is a polyester/plastic layer that gives the film physical stability. Because the emulsion layer is fairly fragile, it needs the plastic base so the film can be handled and processed, yet remain physically strong after processing. Between the emulsion and base layer is an adhesive that simply adheres one layer of the film to another. General radiographic imaging uses double emulsion film with two intensifying screens. The two primary factors affecting speed or sensitivity of radiographic film are the size of silver halide crystals in the emulsion and the number of silver halide crystals. Film manufacturers manipulate film speed by manipulating these two factors. When the number or size of the silver halide crystals increases, the film sensitivity or speed increases.

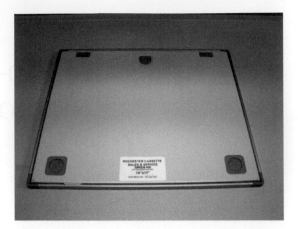

Figure 2.1. X-ray rare earth film cassette.

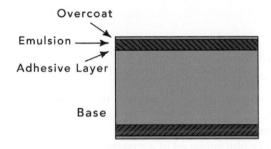

Figure 2.2. Diagram of x-ray film layers.

Film contrast is the ability of radiographic film to provide a certain level of image contrast. High contrast film demonstrates more black and white areas, whereas low contrast film shows shades of gray. Exposure latitude is closely related to film contrast. Film speed, contrast, and latitude are graphically demonstrated in a film's characteristic or sensitometric curve. **Sensitometry** is the study of the relationship between radiation exposure and the amount of density produced. Every film has a different curve.

Intensifying Screens

A **radiographic intensifying screen** is a device that changes the energy of the x-ray beam into a visible light (Fig. 2.3).

This process is called **luminescence**. Intensifying screens show a particular kind of luminescence called **fluorescence**, which means the phosphor is stimulated to emit light only when struck by x-rays. The use of an intensifying screen greatly reduces radiation exposure to technical staff and to the patient. Radiographic intensifying screens generally consist of four basic layers: the protective coating, the phosphor, the reflective or absorbing layer,

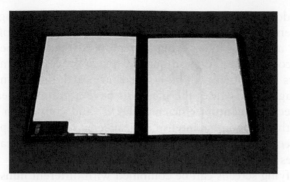

Figure 2.3.   Opened film cassette displaying intensifying screens.

and the base. Today the most common phosphor material is composed of some element from the rare earth group of elements. Rare earth elements are those that range in atomic number from 57 to 71 on the periodic table of the elements.[3] They are called rare earth elements because they are rather difficult and expensive to extract from the earth. Rare earth elements absorb more x-rays, change the x-rays to visible light more efficiently, and result in improved recorded detail when compared to calcium tungstate, the old mainstay phosphor used in intensifying screens until the early 1970s.[2]

The layer of the intensifying screen closest to the film is the protective coating. The active layer of the intensifying screen is the phosphor, which emits light during stimulation by x-rays. The next layer is either the reflective layer or the absorbing layer and is located between the phosphor and the base. Manufacturers will use one or the other but not both. The reflective layer is made of a shiny substance that is either magnesium oxide or titanium dioxide. The phosphor layer emits light with equal intensity in all directions when struck by radiation, and the reflective layer reflects all light toward the film. If the absorbing layer is used, it consists of a light absorbing dye that absorbs the light emitted by the phosphor.[3] The base layer serves as a mechanical support for the active phosphor layer and is made of polyester or high-grade cardboard because it is flexible and chemically inert. The emitted light interacts with the x-ray film to form a latent image. The latent image cannot be seen or detected until it becomes visible by chemical processing. Approximately 30% of the x-rays striking a radiographic intensifying screen interact with the screen.

Spectral emission refers to the color of light produced by a particular intensifying screen. The spectral emission of rare earth intensifying screen phosphors is either a visible blue or green light. Lanthanum oxybromide (LaOBr) emits blue light and gadolinium oxysulfide (Gd_2O_2S) emits green light.[3] X-ray film emulsion is developed to be sensitive to a specific color of light so the light emitted by the intensifying screen should match the film. **Spectral sensitivity** refers to the color of light to which a particular film is most sensitive. It is very important to choose and match the spectral sensitivity of the film with the spectral emission of the intensifying screen. This is called **spectral matching.** Mismatching of film and screens based on spectral emission and sensitivity sharply reduces the speed of the system.

The three most important characteristics of radiographic intensifying screens not affected by the operator of the radiographic system are screen speed, image noise, and spatial resolution. **Screen speed** is a relative number used to describe the efficiency of conversion of x-rays into usable light. The properties that control speed are phosphor thickness, dye, crystal size, and the concentration of phosphor crystal. A thicker phosphor layer, larger phosphor crystals, and higher crystal concentration results in higher screen speed. Light absorbing dyes are added to some phosphors to control the spread of light, which improves **spatial resolution**. Remember spatial resolution is simply the amount of detail in an image. The conditions that affect the intensifying screen speed that the operator of the radiographic system can control are radiation quality, image processing, and temperature.[2]

Image noise occurs more often with high-speed rare earth intensifying screens and high kVp techniques. **Image noise** causes the image to have a grainy appearance and reduces image contrast. **Detective quantum efficiency** (DQE) and **conversion efficiency** (CE) are higher with rare earth radiographic intensifying screens. **DQE** is the percentage of x-rays absorbed by the screen and **CE** is the amount of light emitted for each x-ray absorbed. The higher CE causes the image noise in the higher-speed screens.

Rare earth intensifying screens can be combined with different films to provide varying relative speeds. Relative screen speeds of 200–1200 are available, but if the 1,200 speed system is used, the image may be degraded due to **quantum mottle**, a principal component of image noise, which appears as a grainy, salt-and-pepper-appearing image. A relative speed of 400 is recommended for general radiography to provide a good-quality image. Film-screen and digital imaging artifacts are covered in detail in chapter 5.

Common Principles of Film-Screen and Digital Radiography

There are many similarities and differences between digital radiographic imaging and film-screen radiography. The DR panel, the CR cassette, and the film-screen cassette are image receptors. CR, indirect DR, and film-screen use phosphors to capture the incident x-ray energy and convert to light. The rare earth intensifying screens are made with rare earth elements and some of the older indirect conversion detectors use photodiodes coated with a rare earth scintillator. DQE is an important factor for film-screen, CR, and DR imaging. Image noise is a concern for both digital and film-screen methods of imaging. The spatial resolution for film-screen imaging is superior to digital imaging but contrast resolution with digital imaging systems is better than film-screen.

For both film-screen and digital, the image quality is greatly affected by geometric factors. Source to image distance (**SID**), object image distance (**OID**), and focal spot size affect the sharpness of both the film-screen image and the digital image. Improper alignment of the x-ray tube, the anatomic region to be imaged, and the film-screen cassette or digital detector distorts the shape of the image for both film-screen and digital. The basic radiographic principles learned for film-screen still apply to digital imaging.

Using a technique chart to set the appropriate technical factors (kVp and mAs) for the anatomic part being imaged is critical. Selecting the appropriate anatomic part on the DR console is equally critical for digital imaging to ensure the appropriate computer algorithm for the area of interest is chosen. A grid is equally important to both film-screen and digital imaging in absorbing backscatter radiation to improve the quality of the image.

Digital imaging is faster and there are fewer retakes due to technique settings because it has wider exposure latitude than film-screen imaging. This means the ability to window/level a digital image to adjust the brightness and contrast reduces retakes. There are fewer images taken to display bone and soft tissue with digital because the digital image can be manipulated on the computer to visualize both. Digital is the wave of the future and film-screen imaging will become more obsolete as time passes. But for now, film-screen imaging is still a major part of veterinary imaging.

The Radiographic System 3

Basic Component Overview

The basic components of a radiographic system are a dual focus rotating anode x-ray tube, table, generator, and method of capturing the image. The primary factors involved in producing an image, whether it is with a film-screen or digital system, are source-image distance (SID), milliamperage (mA), exposure time, and kilovoltage (kVp). With a short SID, there will be more distortion of the appearance of the anatomic region of interest and conversely, with a longer SID, there is less distortion. The typical SID is 40–44 inches for most small animal radiographic units (Fig. 3.1).

X-ray Tube

Some dental and portable x-ray units use a single focus stationary or fixed anode x-ray tube because high tube current and power are not necessary (Fig. 3.2).

A general-purpose radiographic system requires a dual focus rotating anode x-ray tube to produce high-intensity x-ray beams in a short time.[2] The dual focus rotating anode x-ray tube consists of a glass or metal electronic vacuum tube containing two electrodes, the negatively charged tungsten cathode or filament and the positively charged rotating anode or target (Fig. 3.3).

In a dual focus x-ray tube, the cathode consists of two tungsten filaments, one filament for small focus and one for the large focus, both embedded in a negatively charged focusing cup (Fig. 3.4).

The focusing cup is made of nickel.[3] Only one filament can be energized during a single exposure. The small filament is used when better spatial resolution is needed for imaging smaller parts like the bones of the head or smaller extremities. The large filament is used

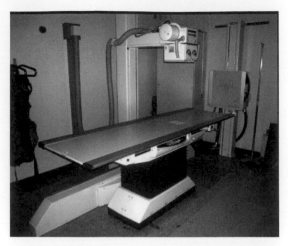

Figure 3.1. X-ray tube head and X-ray table. Image courtesy of D. L. Barber, DVM.

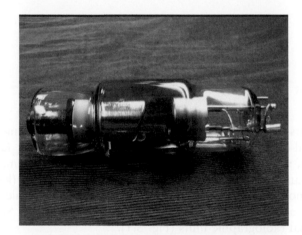

Figure 3.2. Fixed anode single focus x-ray tube in a glass envelope. Image courtesy of D. L. Barber, DVM.

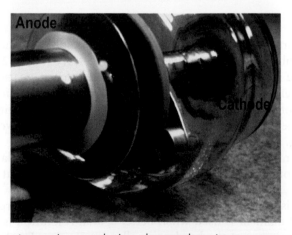

Figure 3.3. Dual focus rotating anode x-ray tube in a glass envelope. Image courtesy of D. L. Barber, DVM.

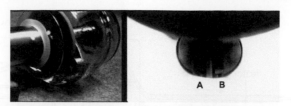

Figure 3.4. Dual focus rotating anode x-ray tube. A, large focus; B, small focus. Image courtesy of D. L. Barber, DVM.

for imaging larger parts like the thorax, abdomen, spine, pelvis, or extremities measuring over 10 cm in thickness.

Prior to developing the rotating anode, manufacturers initiated a design to allow a larger target area to be heated while maintaining a small focal spot by angling the target. Diagnostic x-ray tubes have target angles varying from 5 to 15 degrees. This design is known as the line-focus principle. By angling the target, the effective area of the target is much smaller than the actual area of electron interaction. Due to this design, the radiation intensity on the cathode side of the x-ray field is higher than on the anode side. The x-rays making up the useful beam are emitted from a depth in the target toward the anode side and must travel through a greater thickness of target material than the x-rays emitted in the cathode direction. Because they are emitted through the heel of the target, there is more absorption. This is called the anode heel effect.[2,9,15] The smaller the focal spot, the larger the heel effect. The difference in the intensity of the beam can vary as much as 45%. It is important to keep this fact in mind when imaging patients where there is a significant difference in tissue thickness, like in the abdomen. The cranial abdomen should be positioned on the cathode side of the x-ray tube and the caudal abdomen on the anode side. You can determine which side is the cathode or anode by looking on the protective housing where the cables connect to the x-ray tube. Sometimes it will state anode and cathode but most of the time there will be a + (positive-anode) and − (negative-cathode) marked on the connectors.

When the technician presses the prep or rotor button on the console, the selected filament current will heat the filament and the anode target will start rotating. The outer-shell electrons of the filament atoms are boiled off and ejected from the filament in a process called **thermionic emission**. The outer-shell electrons form into an electron cloud called a space charge in the focus cup. When the exposure button is pressed the kVp setting is applied across the tube from cathode to anode so the highly negatively charged cathode repels the negatively charged electrons away from the cathode as the highly positively charged anode attracts the electrons to the target. This stream of negatively charged electrons is called the **tube current** and is measured in milliamperes (mA).

These negatively charged electrons can create three types of interactions with the target's atoms. As the electrons strike the anode target, they transfer their kinetic energy to the target atoms and are converted to heat. Interestingly, 99% of the electrons are converted to heat and only 1% are converted to x-rays[3] (Fig. 3.5).

The first interaction occurs when projected electrons interact with the target's outer-shell electrons, causing them to rise to an excited higher energy level, but do not transfer enough energy to ionize or remove an orbital electron from an atom. The continuous excitation and return of outer-shell electrons produces most of the heat generated in an x-ray tube anode. The anode disperses the heat to the glass or metal envelope and to the insulating oil surrounding the x-ray tube.

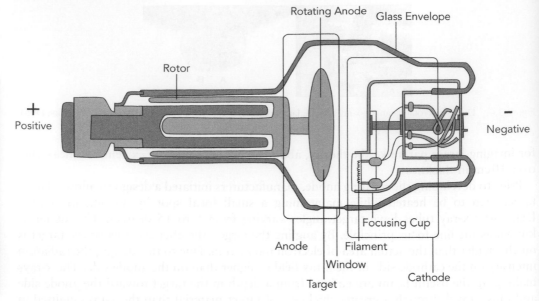

Figure 3.5.   Rotating anode x-ray tube diagram.

Another type of interaction produces characteristic radiation. Characteristic radiation is produced if the negative electron interacts strongly enough with a target atom's inner-shell electron to remove it from the atom. An outer-shell electron automatically replaces the void created by the removal of the inner-shell electron and emits x-rays in the process.

The first two interactions between negatively charged electrons and the x-ray tube's target atoms produce heat and characteristic radiation. A third type of interaction, **Bremsstrahlung interaction,** occurs when the negatively charged electron loses it kinetic energy as it passes through a target atom close enough to the nucleus to come under the influence of its electrical field. This electrical field is very strong because the nucleus contains many protons and the distance between the nucleus and the negatively charged electrons is small. Bremmsstrahlung interactions are also referred to as braking radiation, because as the electron goes by the nucleus, it slows and changes direction. The loss of kinetic energy creates an x-ray emission. Bremmsstrahlung interactions produce most x-ray interactions in the diagnostic energy range of 30–150 kVp.[2,3]

Lastly, there is a window in the glass or metal envelope of the x-ray tube that allows the emitted useful x-ray beam to exit the tube head, then enter and exit the patient, striking the film-screen cassette located in the Bucky tray or DR flat panel.

Fluoroscopy

Fluoroscopy is a special radiographic technique used in specialty practices where an x-ray tube is mounted beneath an x-ray table and coupled with a special unit called an **image intensifier** to produce dynamic or real-time imaging of body functions (Fig. 3.6).

Thomas Edison invented the fluoroscope in 1896.

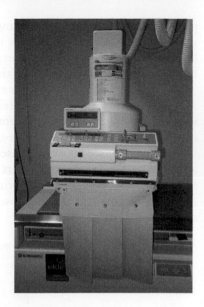

Figure 3.6. Fluoroscopic image intensifier.

An image intensifier is the electronic unit that contains an x-ray image-intensifier tube. The tube components are contained in either a glass or metal envelope that will maintain a vacuum. It intercepts the x-ray beam after it has passed through a patient via an input phosphor made of cesium iodide (CsI), which converts the x-ray beam into a high-intensity visible light image. The input phosphor is generally coupled directly with a television-camera tube to display real-time imaging studies on a video monitor.[2,3,15] The image-intensifying unit also has the ability to record imaging. If a clinician observes something of interest, a permanent image can be taken during the study either via **spot film** or digital image. Depending upon the age of the equipment, there may be a slot in the front of the image intensifier to contain a film-screen cassette, a function button to initiate video recording possibly by VCR or some other means of image capture, or the unit may have the capability to record by taking digital images, singularly, or numerous frames per second. Fluoroscopic imaging is invaluable when used for gastric studies or checking for a collapsing trachea. It is also used for myelography, cystourethrography, and vascular studies. Care must be taken when using this modality because the radiation exposure is higher due to the x-ray beam being emitted for longer lengths of time. Collimation and choosing the correct exposure parameters are imperative when operating fluoroscopic equipment. When the equipment is installed, the service engineer will preprogram the parameters incorporating the type of study with patient size. It is the responsibility of the operator to choose the correct selection and to collimate as closely as possible to the area of interest during the study to reduce exposure to the patient and personnel as well as improve the quality of the image by reducing scatter radiation.

Secondary or Scatter Radiation

The primary beam and secondary or scatter radiation are the two types of radiation responsible for exposing film or a DR panel. The primary beam exits the x-ray tube and passes through the patient unchanged and is recorded on the film or DR panel below. The secondary or scatter radiation is the result of a redirection of part of the primary x-ray beam so the film or DR array is exposed unrelated to the body part. It causes a generalized fog that degrades the quality of the image recorded on film or DR.

To reduce the effects of scatter radiation, collimators and grids are the primary options. A collimator is located immediately below the x-ray tube window and consists of a set of shutters to limit the primary beam as it exits the tube. It also contains a light source that is reflected off of a mirror in the unit and projected onto the table below (Fig. 3.7).

The light source allows the user to see the area being exposed so the shutters can be adjusted as close to the body part to be imaged as possible. Collimation will regulate the size of the area exposed by the primary beam, which results in decreased patient exposure, decreased scatter radiation exposure to holders restraining the patient, and an improved quality image (Fig. 3.8).

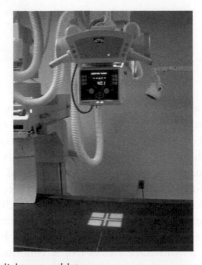

Figure 3.7.   Collimator reflecting light onto tabletop.

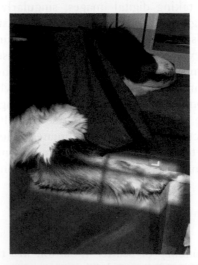

Figure 3.8.   Collimator light centered on left radius ulna. Image courtesy of A. Reid Tyson, DVM.

Grids

A grid is a device constructed with a series of thin linear strips of alternating lead and aluminum designed to absorb scatter radiation before it hits either film or DR array. The grid ratio is the ratio of the height of a grid's lead strips to the distance between them. The higher the ratio, the more efficient the grid is in removing scatter radiation. Typical grid ratios are 5:1, 8:1, 10:1, 12:1, and 16:1. The grid ratio will be imprinted on the grid (Fig. 3.9).

A 300 mA and above machine would typically have a 12:1 grid though some older veterinary units use an 8:1 grid. A grid will absorb 20–30% of the primary beam and 80–90% of scatter radiation so it is necessary to increase technique to compensate when using grid compared to a nongrid technique. It is also imperative the x-ray tube be centered to the grid to prevent grid lines from appearing on the radiographic image or create an artifact called grid cutoff if using film-screen imaging (Fig. 3.10).

Some DR vendors do not support purchasing a grid with their systems, but remember DR arrays are more sensitive to scatter radiation than film-screen systems. Some DR systems have removable grids to allow imaging with and without a grid.

The practitioner should consider purchasing a grid, particularly if the practice is a specialty practice where the imaging caseload is higher and more specialized imaging

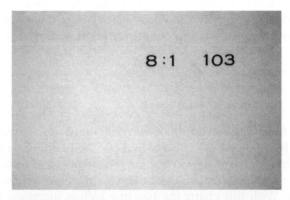

Figure 3.9. Grid ratio imprint from grid surface.

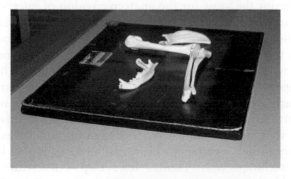

Figure 3.10. Grid on tabletop demonstrating collimation and centering. Image courtesy Jeryl C. Jones, DVM.

procedures are performed, like myelography. If the imaging caseload is low and the typical small animal patient weighs less than 50 lbs, it may not be practical to purchase a system with a grid. This perspective would also apply to a practice using a film-screen system; many small animal practices choose not to use a grid.

Milliamperage and Kilovoltage

When making an x-ray exposure, milliampere seconds (mAs) and kilovolt peak (kVp) are the two exposure factors that determine quantity and quality, respectively, of the x-ray beam. Kilovolt peak controls beam quality and penetrability. A higher-quality x-ray beam is one with higher energy. Kilovolt peak also controls contrast. Lower kVp ranges produce a short scale or high contrast image, which is appropriate for extremity, headwork, abdominal, spine, and pelvic imaging. The higher kVp ranges produce a long scale or low contrast image used mostly for imaging the thorax. With high kVp there is more potential for scatter radiation.

The milliampere station selected determines not only the number of x-rays produced but also the focal spot used. The small focal spot should be used for imaging of the head and extremities if the measurement of the anatomic region is 10 cm or below. For older x-ray generators, 50, 100, 150, and 200 mA stations will generally utilize the small focal spot. The 200 mA station will also utilize the large focal spot on most generators. For thicker anatomic regions like the thorax, abdomen, spine, and pelvis, use a higher mA station and the large focal spot to increase quantity and decrease exposure time. Remember mA × exposure time = mAs; mAs controls radiation quantity, optical density, and patient dose.

Technique Chart

A technique chart is a table with predetermined settings that allow the technician to select the best exposure factors based on the thickness of tissue of the anatomic part being imaged. The two main types of technique charts are variable kVp/fixed mAs and fixed kVp/variable mAs.

For imaging the small animal patient, the author favors a form of the variable kVp/fixed mAs technique chart. With this chart, the baseline kVp is increased by 2 kVp for every 1 cm increase in thickness for patients weighing below 80 lbs; increase 3 kVp per cm for patients weighing 80–100 lbs; and 4 kVp for every cm for patients weighing greater than 100 lbs. The mAs remains the same for the anatomic region of interest[15] (Fig. 3.11).

It is important to use a baseline kVp for each anatomic region that will best visualize the tissue. For example, for extremities, headwork, spine, and abdominal imaging, the kVp settings should be in the 50–80 kVp range. If you have a larger canine patient abdomen, you may have to go to 85 or 90 kVp and/or adjust your mAs in the higher measurement settings to help compensate for the thicker tissue. If using DR or rare earth speed film-screen, it is particularly important to use an adequate mAs setting to prevent quantum mottle, an artifact caused by using too little mAs. A fixed kVp/variable mAs technique chart does not work well in veterinary medicine due to motion caused by too long of an exposure. In veterinary medicine technique chart formulation, Santes' Rule is very popular to use to formulate a technique chart. [Santes' Rule: kVp = (2 × tissue thickness) + FFD + Grid Factor[10,15,21] (Table 3.1).]

Technique Chart

Feline, Canine Thorax

Measurement cm.	kVp	kVp	mA	Time	mAS	mAs
3-4	48		300	1/60	5.0	
5-6	50		300	1/60	5.0	
7-8	52		300	1/60	5.0	
9-10	54		300	1/60	5.0	
11	56		300	1/60	5.0	
12	58		300	1/60	5.0	
13	58		300	1/60	5.0	
14	60		300	1/60	5.0	
15	62		300	1/60	5.0	
16-17	64		300	1/60	5.0	
17-18	68		300	1/60	5.0	
19-20	70		300	1/60	5.0	
21	72		300	1/60	5.0	
22	74		300	1/60	5.0	
23	76		300	1/60	5.0	
24	78		300	1/60	5.0	
25	80		300	1/60	5.0	
27-28	82		300	1/60	5.0	
29-30	84		300	1/60	5.0	

Feline, Canine Abdomen

Measurement	kVp	kVp	mA	Time	mAS	mAS
3-4	44		300	1/30	10.0	
5-6	46		300	1/30	10.0	
7-8	48		300	1/30	10.0	
9-10	50		300	1/30	10.0	
11-12	52		300	1/30	10.0	
13	55		300	1/30	10.0	
14	57		300	1/30	10.0	
15	57		300	1/30	10.0	
16	60		300	1/30	10.0	
17	63		300	1/30	10.0	
18	66		300	1/30	10.0	
19	68		300	1/30	10.0	
20	70		300	1/30	10.0	
21	73		300	1/30	10.0	
22	75		300	1/30	10.0	
23	77		300	1/30	10.0	
24	78		300	1/30	10.0	
25	81		300	1/30	10.0	
26	85		300	1/30	10.0	
27-28	88		300	1/30	10.0	

Feline and Canine Extremity and Headwork

Measurement	kVp	kVp	mA	Time	mAS	mAS
2-3	42		100	1/30	3.3	
4	44		100	1/30	3.3	
5	46		100	1/20	5.0	
6	48		100	1/20	5.0	
7	48		100	1/20	5.0	
8	50		100	1/20	5.0	
9	52		100	1/20	5.0	
10	54		100	1/12	8.3	
11	56		200	1/20	10.0	
12	58		200	1/20	10.0	
13	60		200	1/20	10.0	
14	62		200	1/20	10.0	
15	64		200	1/20	10.0	
16	66		200	1/20	10.0	
17	70		200	1/20	10.0	
18	72		200	1/20	10.0	
19	76		200	1/20	10.0	
20	77		200	1/20	10.0	
21	78		200	1/20	10.0	
22	80		200	1/20	10.0	

Feline, Canine – Spine and Pelvis

Measurement cm.	kVp	kVp	mA	Time	mAS	mAS
3-4	50		300	1/30	10.0	
5-6	52		300	1/30	10.0	
7-8	54		300	1/30	10.0	
9-10	56		300	1/30	10.0	
11	58		300	1/30	10.0	
12	60		300	1/30	10.0	
13	64		300	1/30	10.0	
14	66		300	1/30	10.0	
15	66		300	1/30	10.0	
16	68		300	1/30	10.0	
17-18	70		300	1/30	10.0	
19-20	72		300	1/30	10.0	
21	74		300	1/30	10.0	
22	74		300	1/30	10.0	
23	76		300	1/30	10.0	
24	76		300	1/30	10.0	
25	78		300	1/30	10.0	
26	80		300	1/30	10.0	
27-28	82		300	1/30	10.0	

Figure 3.11. Sample Technique Chart.

Table 3.1.   Variable kVp technique chart formulation guide.[10,15,21]

Step 1.

If using a film-screen imaging system, have your darkroom processor serviced so image quality won't be affected by film-processing errors and issues.

Make sure the x-ray film matches the intensifying screens in your film cassettes. Remember **spectral emission** refers to the color of light produced by a particular intensifying screen. X-ray film emulsion is developed to be sensitive to a specific color of light, so the light emitted by the intensifying screen should match the film. **Spectral sensitivity** refers to the color of light to which a particular film is most sensitive. It is very important to choose and match the spectral sensitivity of the film with the spectral emission of the intensifying screen. This is called **spectral matching**. Mismatching of film and screens based on spectral emission and sensitivity sharply reduces the speed of the system.

Choose a mature dog weighing approximately 40–50 pounds that is not overweight or underweight. It is preferable for the dog to be under anesthesia.

Step 2. Choose your mAs settings.

Remember most of your patients are awake or sedated, so motion can be a primary cause of blurred images. If your x-ray machine has more than one mA station, choose a lower mA station (100 or 150 mA) for tabletop extremity and headwork to take advantage of using a small focal spot. For table Bucky extremities (over 10 cm thickness), thorax, abdomen, pelvis, and spine, use the highest mA station (300 mA) to allow choosing shorter exposure times.

Remember **mA × time = mAs**. Example: 300 mA × 1/120 = 2.5 mAs or 100 mA × 1/40 = 2.5 mAs.

Recommendation for Par (medium 200) speed intensifying screens:

Tabletop (no grid) extremity or headwork: 2.5 mAs.

Thorax: 5 mAs.

Abdomen: 7.5 mAs.

Spine/Pelvis: 10 mAs.

Step 3. Choose your initial kVp: Use Santes' Rule to find the initial kVp to go along with the suggested mAs setting.

Santes' Rule: kVp = (2 × tissue thickness) + FFD (focal film distance) + grid factor.

Focal film distance is usually set to 40 inches in veterinary medicine. Grids require more radiation to achieve the same exposure, so if you are using a grid, extra kVp will have to be added. 8:1 ratio grids are most commonly used in veterinary medicine. If you do not use a grid, use 0 (zero) for the grid factor.

5:1 grid—add 6–8 kVp.

8:1 grid—add 8–10 kVp.

12:1 grid—add 10–15 kVp.

Place the patient in a lateral recumbent position. Measure the patient's cranial abdomen over the thickest point, using a caliper. For example, the patient measured 14 cm. The FFD is 40 inches and the table Bucky has an 8:1 ratio grid. Using Santes' Rule, the initial kVp would be 78 kVp = (2 × 14) + 40 + 10.

Table 3.1. (*Continued*)

Step 4. Make the exposure.

Using our example, the technical factors used were 78 kVp and 7.5 mAs. If the radiograph is good quality, you have the starting point for a technique chart for the abdomen. If not, then the technique will need to be adjusted by the kVp 15% rule.

If the radiograph is too dark, decrease the kVp by 15%. If the radiograph is too light, increase the kVp by 15%.

If the technique is still off, keep increasing or decreasing the kVp in 5% increments until you are satisfied with the result.

Step 5. Make the technique chart. Start with the adjusted technique and interpolate to find the values of kVp for other measurements following the rules below:

Subtract 2 kVp from the original kVp for each cm decrease from the original measurement.

Add 2 kVp to the original kVp for each cm increase from the original measurement up to 80 kVp.

Add 3 kVp for each cm increase that places the kVp above 80 up to 100.

Add 4 kVp for each cm increase that places the kVp above 100.

Step 6. Repeat the above process to make a technique chart for each different study (abdomen, thorax, extremity, pelvis/spine).

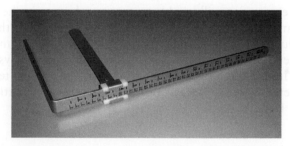

Figure 3.12. Caliper measuring instrument.

Factors affecting a technique chart are SID (source-image distance) or FFD (focal film distance), beam filtration, and grid/nongrid. A technique chart is a necessity for both film-screen radiography and DR to prevent overexposure to the patient and holders and to prevent DR artifacts like quantum mottle and fogging. Please remember technique charts will only work if you use them.

It is necessary to use a caliper to measure for each view. A **caliper** is an L-shaped measuring instrument with centimeter markings, used to measure the thickness of the anatomic region of interest (Fig. 3.12).

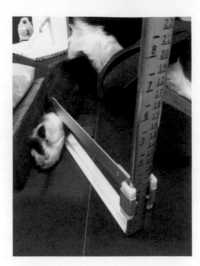

Figure 3.13.   Caliper measurement of canine carpus. Image courtesy of A. Reid Tyson, DVM.

Always measure the patient over the thickest part of the area of interest **after** the patient has been positioned (Fig. 3.13).

Recording technical factors for each view of a radiographic exam on every patient is a good practice to evaluate the technique chart so changes can be made, as needed. Recording technical factors will also help reduce unnecessary repeat exposures on follow-up patient exams (Fig. 3.14).

For example, the veterinarian will be able to monitor changes in the patient's condition by noting minute changes in lung patterns or heart size or follow-up thorax imaging. The practice will also reduce radiation exposure to the patient, holders, and to the DR array, if using a digital system, by reducing retakes. If using a film-screen system, the technique sheet can be inserted into the film jacket for storage. If using DR, the technical factors can be recorded on a patient log. It is very easy to either insert this information into a computer log or a handwritten log.

Overexposure vs. Underexposure

Similar principles apply to both film-screen systems and DR systems when addressing overexposure and underexposure issues. The technique chart plays a critical role to both systems. If the patient is emaciated or has a lot of gas in the stomach and intestines, the kVp may need to be decreased; conversely, if the patient is an obese or muscular animal, both kVp and mAs may need to be increased to produce a quality image. Quantum mottle or noise is caused by underexposure, that is, too little mAs with either system. With DR, window and leveling can improve the image some but with film-screen systems, the best option is to retake the film with an adjusted technique. The veterinary technician may have to investigate why the image on the film appears underexposed. It may not be the technique chart. If the darkroom chemistry is becoming exhausted, the image on the film may appear underexposed (Table 3.2).

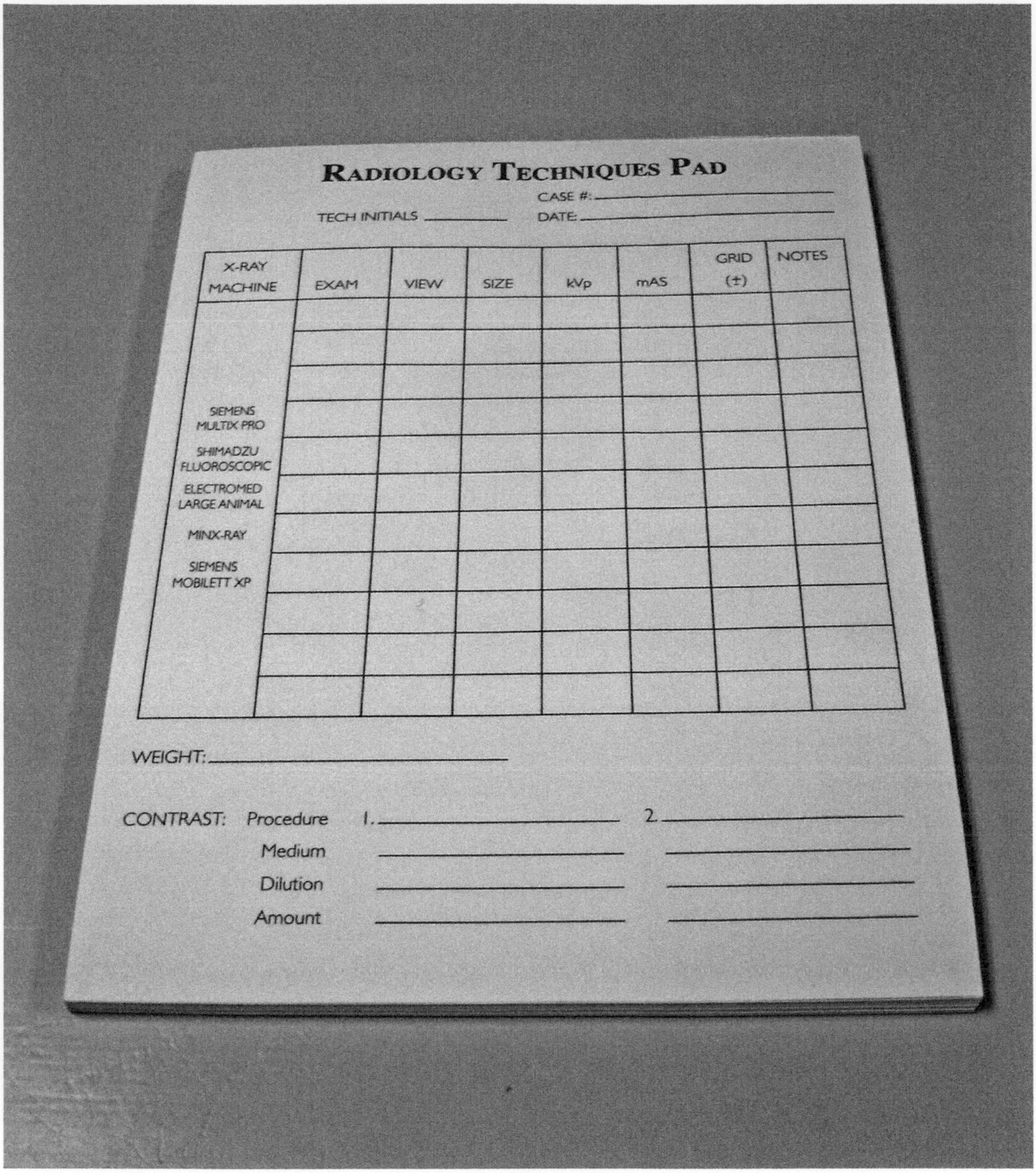

Figure 3.14.   Example of radiographic technique recording sheet.

Patient Log

Every practice should maintain a daily patient imaging log, either hardcopy or electronically. The log should consist of a listing of the date, client/animal's name, species, breed, patient exam, and possibly the views or number of views taken. Some patient logs will include the technical factors used if this information is not recorded elsewhere in the patient's radiographic film jacket or patient medical record. A radiology patient daily log is required in some states as a license requirement (Fig. 3.15).

Table 3.2. Evaluating the Improperly Exposed Radiograph. Table Courtesy of Matt Wright, DVM, DACVR Animal Insides

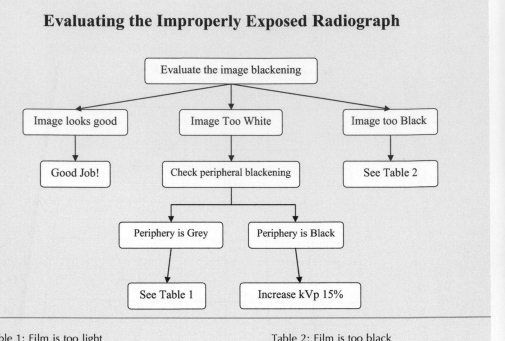

Evaluating the Improperly Exposed Radiograph

- Evaluate the image blackening
  - Image looks good
    - Good Job!
  - Image Too White
    - Check peripheral blackening
      - Periphery is Grey
        - See Table 1
      - Periphery is Black
        - Increase kVp 15%
  - Image too Black
    - See Table 2

Table 1: Film is too light	Table 2: Film is too black
Common Causes	**Common Causes**
Insufficient Technique: Double the mAs	Excessive Technique
Used the wrong technique chart	Decrease mAs by 50%
Measured Incorrectly	Decrease kVp by 15%
X-ray tube height is too high	Double Exposure
X-ray tube not aligned with grid	X-ray tube height is too low
Less Common Causes: Processor Problems	**Less Common Causes: Processor Problems**
Developer Exhausted	Developer too strong
Developer Diluted	Developer temperature too high
Inadequate developer replenishment	Processor timer malfunction
Developer Temperature too low	**Less Common Causes; Darkroom Problems**
Processor Timer Malfunction	Light Fog
Rare Causes:	Safety Light Malfunction
X-ray machine miscalibration	**Rare Causes**
X-ray tube failure	X-ray machine timer malfunction
X-ray machine timer malfunction	X-ray machine miscalibration

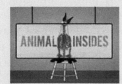

www.animalinsides.com

X-RAY LOG

NUMBER	PATIENT NAME	BREED	DATE	VIEW(S)	AREA OF INTEREST	CM.	KVP	MA	SEC.	MAS	RESULT

Figure 3.15. Example of imaging log.

It is also a very helpful tool with many applications. For example, if a practice is using film-screen imaging, the log can help track how many patients have been imaged between darkroom processor cleanings. Technique charts do not work as efficiently when the darkroom chemistry becomes exhausted. If searching for a particular patient imaging exam to use the same technical factors as the last time because it is a recheck exam for pneumonia, the information can be found quickly, particularly if the practice is using an electronic daily patient log. The log can be set up as a simple Excel spreadsheet workbook.

CHAPTER 3

X-RAY LOG

Figure 4-5. Example of imaging log.

It is also a very helpful tool with many applications. For example, if a practice is using film-screen imaging, the log can help track how many patients have been imaged between darkroom processor cleanings. Technique charts do not work as efficiently when the darkroom chemistry becomes exhausted. If searching for a particular patient imaging exam to use the same technical factors as the last time because it is a recheck exam for pneumonia, the information can be found quickly, particularly if the practice is using an electronic daily print-out log. The log can be set up as a simple Excel spreadsheet workbook.

Darkroom Maintenance and Film Processing

Darkroom Setup

The darkroom is an integral part of any veterinary practice using a film-screen system. Film processing is as important as technique and positioning in making a quality radiograph. Processing the invisible latent image creates the visible manifest image. Processing converts the light-exposed silver ions in the silver halide crystal to microscopic black grains of silver. Following good darkroom maintenance practices is necessary to producing good-quality images. Darkrooms must be free from all outside white-light exposure. The color of the interior walls should be light to reflect the small amount of light available from safelights. The paint should be semi-gloss or flat in texture. Floors should be made of a material that makes them nonslippery when wet in the event of chemical or water spills or leaks inside the darkroom.

The darkroom should be wiped clean daily to minimize artifacts on film by maintaining the cleanest possible conditions in the room. The floor should be mopped with a damp mop. All unnecessary items should be removed from countertops and work surfaces. A clean damp towel should be used to wipe off the processor feed tray and all countertops and work surfaces. If a cassette pass box is present, it should be cleaned daily as well. Hands should be kept clean to minimize fingerprints and handling artifacts. Overhead air vents and safelights should be wiped or vacuumed weekly before other cleaning procedures are performed. The ceiling tiles should be cleaned to prevent flaking on a monthly basis. Eating and drinking in the darkroom should be prohibited. Nothing should be on the countertop except for items used for loading and unloading cassettes because they will collect dust. There should be no shelves above the countertops in the darkroom since these too serve as a site for dust collection.

Manual Film Processing

The manual processing darkroom should have designated dry and wet areas to facilitate keeping the room as clean and clutter-free as possible. The dry area is used to store undeveloped film and film hangers, for loading and unloading film from cassettes, and for placing films on hangers for processing. The wet area will contain the processing tanks and space for drying film post-processing. The processing tank system will consist of a developer, rinse, fixer, and wash tanks. Dry towels should be kept in the darkroom to wipe up spills. Use a timer when manual processing to avoid overdeveloping or underfixing a film.

Film developing is a chemical process, therefore the developer, rinse, fixer, rinse, and wash temperatures should be the same. The optimal developer temperature is 20°C or 68°F for most film types. At 68°F, the developing time should be 5 minutes. Use a thermometer to check the chemistry temperature prior to processing film. Check the manufacturer's instructions for specific details. Using higher than recommended developer temperatures followed by placing the film in too cool fixer will make the film's emulsion swell and thicken unevenly, causing it to slip or fall off the film base, creating a wrinkled or corrugated appearance called reticulation (Fig. 4.1).

Care must be taken when placing a film in or removing a film from the developer tank to prevent scratching the film. Always gently agitate the film when first immersed to remove any air bubbles so the developer solution can reach the film surface.

The next tank is the rinse bath or stop bath. When the film is removed from developer and placed in the rinse bath, gently agitate the film for 30 seconds to remove the developing chemistry to minimize contamination before placing the film in the fixing solution tank. Circulating water works well or a stop bath solution, which is 1.5% acetic acid, can be used. The stop bath solution will quickly stop the action of the developer as well as neutralize the alkali of the developing solution and protect the acidity of the fixing solution.[15]

The fixing solution consists of a fixing agent, an acidifier, a hardener, a preservative, and a solvent. The fixer will clear undeveloped silver crystals from the film, neutralize the developer solution, and shrink and harden the film emulsion. Gently agitate the film for about 15 seconds to avoid streaks and stains on the film when first immersed in the fixing

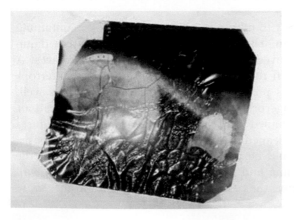

Figure 4.1.   Reticulated x-ray film. Image courtesy of Jeryl C. Jones, DVM.

tank. The fixing time can be determined by the clearing time. The clearing time is the length of time it takes for the film appearance to change from cloudy to clear. This is dependent upon the age and strength of the fixing solution. The fixing solution is exhausted and should be replaced when clearing time exceeds 3 minutes. After the film as cleared, leave in the fixing solution twice as long as the clearing time. If it takes 2 minutes for the film to clear, the total fixing time should be 6 minutes. If the film is not left in the fixing solution long enough or if the fixing solution is too weak, the image on the film will fade and discolor with age.

The next step is to place the film in the wash tank. Some manual darkrooms may have a post-fixer rinse bath set up prior to placing film in the wash tank. If so, gently agitate the film for 30 seconds in the second rinse and then place in the final rinse or wash tank. The wash tank contains circulating water, which will wash away remaining chemicals from the film. The length of time film is left in the wash bath is dependent upon the number of water changes per hour. Typically, films should be washed for about 20 minutes in circulating water in which the flow is 10 times the volume of the tank per hour. If films are left in the wash tank too long, the emulsion will swell and fall off the film base. One reference stated films could be left in the wash tank overnight without permanent damage, but this practice is not recommended. Algae in the wash tank can be controlled by filtering incoming water. Draining and cleaning the water tanks weekly will provide additional protection from algae.

The last step is drying the processed film. After being removed from the wash, films should be hung in a dry place where water can drain off of them either into a sink or tray. It takes approximately 2 hours for film to dry. Film will dry more efficiently in a film dryer, a cabinet that blows warm air over film placed on a rack. It is not recommended to just use a fan to blow air onto the drying film due to the possibility of blowing dust onto the film. A wetting agent bath can be used just after removing the film from the wash to decrease drying time. The film is briefly immersed into a tank containing a commercial wetting agent before being placed in a dryer. After the film has dried, cut off the corners of the film where the hanger attached with scissors or a film corner cutter, and place in the patient's film jacket (Fig. 4.2).

Darkroom chemistry solutions lose strength and volume during use. Replenisher solutions can be added in quantities to restore to proper levels and the product instructions will help with this process. Remember replenisher solutions are not the same as regular solutions and repeated use and time will eventually exhaust darkroom chemistry solutions, even when replenishers are added. Darkroom chemistry solutions should be changed monthly and earlier if the developer solution turns green or brown and/or the clearing time in the fixing bath takes as long as 2–3 minutes. Make sure to clean the chemistry tanks before refilling with fresh chemistry solutions. Water tanks should be drained and cleaned at least weekly to prevent algae from growing. Placing a filter on incoming water will also help eliminate algae. If algae appear, clean the water tanks and the water lines to the tanks with an algaecide or diluted laundry bleach solution.[9,15]

Automatic Film Processing

With automatic x-ray film processing, the sequence consists of developing, where the emulsion swells and the developing chemical changes the silver ions of the exposed crystals into

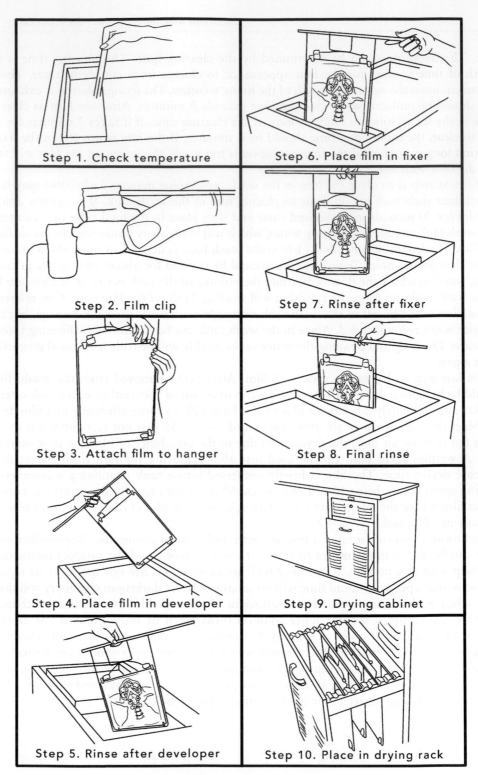

Step 1. Check temperature

Step 2. Film clip

Step 3. Attach film to hanger

Step 4. Place film in developer

Step 5. Rinse after developer

Step 6. Place film in fixer

Step 7. Rinse after fixer

Step 8. Final rinse

Step 9. Drying cabinet

Step 10. Place in drying rack

Figure 4.2. Manual x-ray film processing instructional diagram. Adapted from images from William R. Brawner, DVM.

metallic silver. The next step is fixing, where the silver halide that was not exposed to radiation is dissolved and removed from the emulsion and the gelatin portion of the emulsion is hardened at the same time to make it structurally more sound. The next step is washing any remaining chemicals from the film. Last, the film is transported through the dryer to remove the water used to wash it and to make the film acceptable for handling and viewing (Fig. 4.3).

Automatic Film Processor Maintenance

The x-ray film processor should be cleaned monthly, replacing all of the chemistry, mixing fresh chemistry, and cleaning the water tank and lines. Any worn transport rollers should be replaced during the monthly maintenance. The crossover rollers should be wiped off daily. An automatic processor should be turned on daily (preferably at least five times weekly) and cleanup film processed to replenish the chemistry and keep water flowing through the wash tank and water line. Draining and filling the water tank daily will help prevent the development of algae in the wash tank (Fig. 4.4).

CHAPTER 4

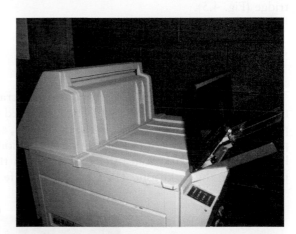

Figure 4.3. Tabletop automatic x-ray film processor.

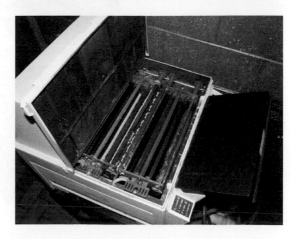

Figure 4.4. Automatic tabletop x-ray film processor crossover rollers.

After the processor warms up to optimal temperature, processing approximately six cleanup films daily will replenish the developer and fixer chemistry, extending its life. If available, you can use out-of-date film for this process. Take three films from your out-of-date film box, expose to white light, and then process. Take another three films from your out-of-date film box and process without exposing to white light. The exposed film should come out black and the unexposed film should be fairly clear, though it may have some fog due to age. You are primarily making sure the developer is turning the background density black and not brown or streaking, signs that the developer needs to be replaced. The film should also be dry, not brittle or sticky, signs of fixer, wash, or dryer issues.

Silver Recovery Cartridges

A silver recovery cartridge should be connected to the processor to filter the used fixer from the processor because the fixer solution contains a high concentration of accumulated silver. Silver is considered a heavy metal, and disposing of it is regulated by local and state agencies. The company that repairs or maintains your processor should check, pick up the silver cartridge when it has reached capacity, and replace with a new silver recovery cartridge (Fig. 4.5).

Safelights

The safelight filters should be checked daily for cracks that may allow white light exposure to film. The spectral sensitivity of film, discussed earlier, also relates to the color of light produced with safelight filters. In the darkroom, safelight filters are placed in safelights to produce a particular color of light for illumination. It is important to use the correct safelight filter in all darkroom safelights based on the spectral sensitivity of the film being processed in the darkroom. The GBX filter is safe for both blue- and green-sensitive films.

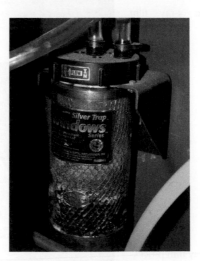

Figure 4.5. Silver recovery cartridge.

GBX simply stands for green/blue x-ray. The Wratten 1A safelight filter is safe for green-sensitive films only and the Wratten 6B safelight filter is safe for blue-sensitive film only.

An incorrect match between the type of safelight filter and the spectral sensitivity of film results in a high incidence of safelight fogging on the film. This fogging appears radiographically as a film with increased density and decreased contrast. Exposed radiographic films are eight times more sensitive to fog than unexposed film. The effect on x-ray film of exposure to the illumination from safelight lamps is referred to post-exposure. The quality of a radiograph may be impaired by unnecessary exposure to safelight illumination, which is the reason for variations in density encountered in routine radiographs and for the lack of brilliancy that is frequently attributed to scattered radiation. If it appears this is a problem in your practice, reduce the intensity of the safelight illumination by using lower wattage bulbs, increase the distance between the safelight lamps and the top of the film-loading counter, or reduce the number safelight lamps in the darkroom.

Film Storage and Handling

Improper storage and handling of x-ray film result in poor radiographs with artifacts that can interfere with patient care. Improper handling or processing can also cause artifacts on the processed radiograph. X-ray film is pressure-sensitive, so rough handling or the imprint of a fingernail is reproduced as an artifact. Creasing the film before processing produces a line artifact. If there is dirt on hands or on the intensifying screens, the result is an artifact that is speckled in appearance. In a dry environment, static electricity can cause characteristic artifacts. During automatic processing, wear or dirt on the transport system causes artifacts. X-ray film is sensitive to the effects of elevated temperature and humidity, especially for long periods of time. Heat reduces contrast and increases fog on the radiograph. Film should be stored away from heat sources, ionizing radiation, and darkroom chemistry storage. Film not in a film bin ideally should be refrigerated. Storage for a year or longer is acceptable if the film is maintained at 50°F. Film should be stored in its original container box and oriented vertically to prevent pressure artifacts on the film (Fig. 4.6).

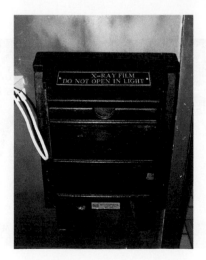

Figure 4.6.   Film bin.

CHAPTER 4

Other potential hazards to film in the darkroom include heat and chemical exposure. Film stored within the darkroom should not be close to any heat source. Like film stored in a refrigerated area, film boxes should be stored vertically, not horizontally, to prevent pressure artifacts on the film. The proper room temperature for storing film is 50–70°F with a relative humidity of 40–60%. Use out-of-date film as clean up film to maintain your processor chemistry replenishment. Processing chemicals must be kept away from film and film-handling areas to prevent exposure and contamination of these areas. Film fogging will occur with age so it is a good practice to use older film first.

Post-processed radiographs should be stored between 60°F and 80°F and between 30% and 50% relative humidity. Radiographs are legally part of the patient's medical record, giving ownership and responsibility for those records to the practice that produced them. Though x-ray film has a safety designation as technically nonflammable, the jackets they are stored in are flammable so films should be stored in a nonsmoking area and on metal shelving to further decrease the fire hazard.

Patient Identification Labeling

Patient information should be imprinted on film prior to processing to provide permanent patient identification. The most prevalent way to imprint the information is to use a photo imprinting device, sometimes referred to as a film ID printer (Fig. 4.7).

Film cassettes can be ordered with a patient ID blocker manufactured. You can also order a regular cassette with intensifying screens and cover a corner on both the front and back intensifying screen with special tape that does not allow the screen crystals to be affected by x-rays. Patient information is printed on a card and the card is placed in a slot on the printer with a corner of the film overlying the card. The printer is closed and a light flashes under the card and imprints the patient information on the film prior to being placed on the entry tray to the processor.

Removable lead letters and numbers that fit into a holder is another method of identifying a patient. The holder is placed on the cassette and exposed to x-rays with the patient during imaging.

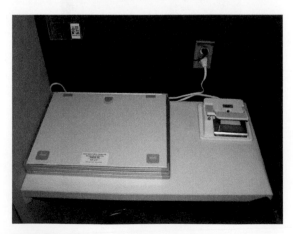

Figure 4.7.   Film ID printer and darkroom counter space.

A less expensive method of permanently imprinting patient information on the film is to use lead impregnated tape. This method is also used prior to exposing the film. The technician writes the identifying information on the tape and then the tape is placed on the cassette prior to the exposure.

Care and Maintenance of Film Cassettes

As discussed earlier, an intensifying screen is a device found in radiographic cassettes that contain phosphors that convert x-ray energy into light, which then exposes the radiographic film. The purpose of intensifying screens is to decrease the radiation dose needed to expose the radiographic film. The screen mounted in the tube side of the cassette is called the front screen and the screen mounted on the opposite side of the cassette is called the back screen.

The care and maintenance of intensifying screens is extremely important because radiographic quality depends in large part on how well the screens are continuously maintained. Dust, hair, or other foreign material is transferred to the screens when the cassette is opened. If left on the screen, it can eventually penetrate the screen surface, leaving a permanent artifact. Regularly clean the intensifying screens with a commercially available antistatic intensifying screen cleaner with gauze pads. Cleaning intensifying screens twice a month is a good practice and will prolong the life of the screen (Fig. 4.8).

Check the cassettes for film-screen contact. Poor film-screen contact degrades recorded detail and is usually seen as a localized area of unsharpness somewhere on the radiographic image. Common causes of poor screen-film contact are worn contact felt; loose, bent, or broken hinges or latches; warped screens resulting from excessive moisture; warped cassette front; sprung or cracked cassette frame; and foreign matter under the screen (Fig. 4.9).

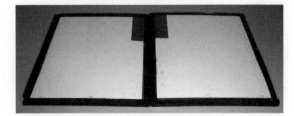

Figure 4.8.　Dirty intensifying screen.

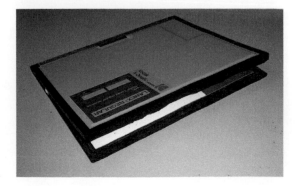

Figure 4.9.　Broken cassette hinges.

A good practical tip is to number your cassettes by writing the cassette number using a permanent black marker on the surface of one of the screens in a corner out of the way. The same number needs to be written on the outside of the cassette. The screen number will show up on images produced with that cassette and will make it easier to test the cassette in question.

The test to check film-screen contact requires a special wire mesh test tool. The wire mesh tool is simply placed on the cassette in question and radiographed using the technical factors 50 kVp at 5 mAs and a SID of 40 inches. The resulting radiograph is then viewed at a distance of about 6 feet to determine whether there are any areas of unsharpness. Areas of poor contact will appear darker, cloudy, or blurred when compared to areas of good contact because of the increased spreading out of the light photons (Fig. 4.10).

Cassettes should be checked frequently to make sure the screens are adhered securely to the cassette; the felt is not worn, allowing light leaks; and the latches and hinges are in good condition (Fig. 4.11).

In an earlier chapter, luminescence was defined as the emission of light from the screen when stimulated by radiation. Intensifying screens may luminesce in two ways, fluorescence or phosphorescence. Fluorescence refers to the ability of phosphors to emit visible light only while exposed to x-rays. Phosphorescence occurs when screen phosphors continue to emit light after the x-ray exposure has stopped. This is also referred to as screen

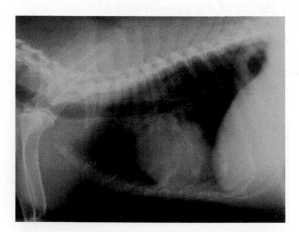

Figure 4.10. Radiographic image depicting poor screen contact. Image courtesy of Jeryl C. Jones, DVM.

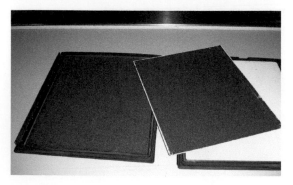

Figure 4.11. Loose intensifying screens.

lag and will cause general overall fogging of the radiographic image and degrading of the scale of contrast in the radiographic image. Screen lag is generally due to old, worn-out screens. To test for lag, make a normal exposure of an object with the cassette empty of any film. Immediately take the cassette to the darkroom and place a film in it, close the cassette, and allow the film to remain in the cassette for 5 minutes. Develop the film in the same manner as a normally exposed radiograph. If the image of the object is transmitted onto the film, then the screens have lag and need to be replaced.

Film-Screen and Digital Imaging Artifacts

An artifact is any unwanted optical density on an image that does not properly show the anatomic area of interest being examined. Artifacts can interfere with visualization of the anatomic region of interest and can lead to misdiagnosis. Artifacts can be controlled when their cause is properly identified.

For x-ray film, the cause can be narrowed down to when an artifact was created. Primarily artifacts can occur when the film is being exposed; when the film is being processed; and when the film is being handled and stored, either before or after processing.

Exposure Artifacts

Common exposure artifacts are unexpected foreign objects (such as dog collars); double exposure; motion; grid cutoff; and quantum mottle. The cause and solution for each artifact is listed in Table 5.1 (see also Figs. 5.1 through 5.4).

Table 5.1. Common exposure artifacts.

Appearance on Radiographic Film	Cause
Unexpected foreign objects	Improper patient preparation—remove collars and leashes
Double exposure	Reuse of cassettes already exposed
Motion	Improper patient movement/restraint
Grid cutoff and grid lines	Improper alignment of x-ray tube to grid. The x-ray tube should be centered to the grid
Quantum mottle	Insufficient mAS. Increase mAs by using a higher mA selection and/or increase length of the exposure. May be necessary to adjust kVp if using a 300 mA generator

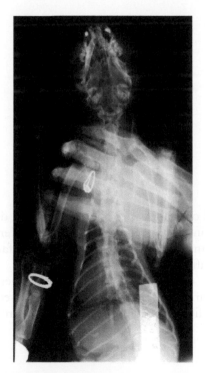

Figure 5.1. Foreign object on patient.

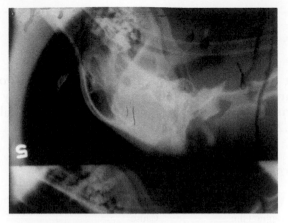

Figure 5.2. Double exposed film.

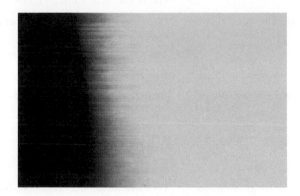

Figure 5.3. Grid cutoff.

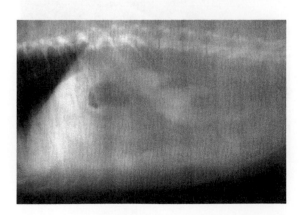

Figure 5.4. Grid lines.

Darkroom Processing Artifacts

Common processing artifacts are guide-shoe marks; pi lines; uniform dull, gray fog; dichroic stain or "curtain" effect; yellow-brown drops on film; milky appearance; greasy appearance; and wrinkled or corrugated appearance when manual processing, called reticulation (Table 5.2; Figs. 5.5 through 5.8).

Table 5.2.   Common processing artifacts.

Appearance on Radiographic Film	Cause
Guide-shoe marks	Improper position or springing of guide shoes in turn-around assembly
Pi lines	Dirt or chemical stains on rollers
Sharp increase or decrease in optical density	Dirty or warped rollers, which can leave sludge deposits on film
Uniform dull, gray fog	Improper or inadequate processing chemistry
Dichroic stain or "curtain" effect	Improper squeezing of processing chemicals from film
Small circular patterns of increased optical density	Pressure caused by irregular or dirty rollers
Yellow-brown drops on film	Oxidized developer
Milky appearance	Unreplenished fixer
Greasy appearance	Inadequate washing
Reticulation (manual processing)—wrinkled or corrugated appearance	Excessive temperature difference between developer and fixer or developer and clearing agent. Check chemistry temperature prior to processing

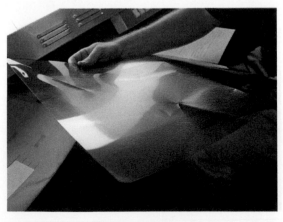

Figure 5.5.   Depicts how crescent or kink marks are made. Image courtesy of Jeryl C. Jones, DVM.

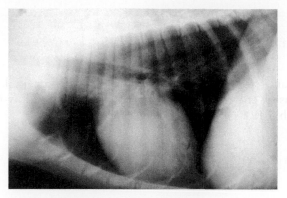

Figure 5.6. Post-processed image with crescent mark.

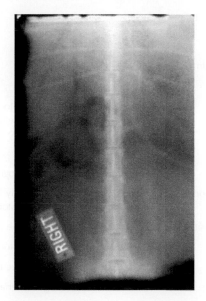

Figure 5.7. White light leak. Image courtesy of Jeryl C. Jones, DVM.

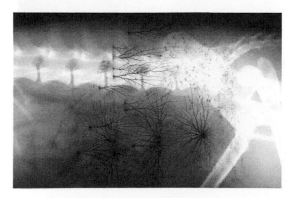

Figure 5.8. Static artifact.

53

Film Storage Artifacts

Common handling and storage artifacts are fog; pressure or kink marks; streaks of increased optical density; crown, tree, and smudge static; and yellow-brown stains (Table 5.3; Figs. 5.9 through 5.12).

Digital Imaging Artifacts

Computed radiography and direct radiography systems have unique artifact patterns as a result of errors in the systems and inadequate technique, collimation, etc. Some of the

Table 5.3.   Common handling and storage artifacts.

Appearance on Radiographic Film	Cause
Fog	The temperature or humidity is too high The film bin is inadequately shielded from radiation The safelight is too bright, or too close to the processing tray, or has an improper filter Expired film Loaded film cassette left in radiographic room
Pressure or kink marks (half-moon marks)	The film is improperly or roughly handled The film is stacked too high in storage and not stored vertically
Streaks of increased optical density	There are white-light leaks in the darkroom or cassette
Crown, tree, and smudge static	The temperature or humidity is too low
Yellow-brown stains	Thiosulfate is left on the film due to inadequate washing
Unidentifiable objects on image	Hair, dirt, flakes of foreign material on intensifying screen

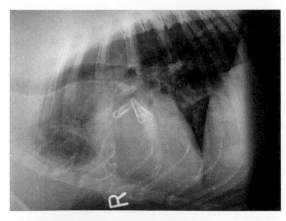

Figure 5.9.   Foreign object in cassette.

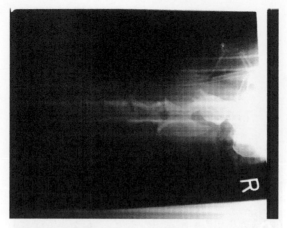

Figure 5.10. Guide-shoe marks.

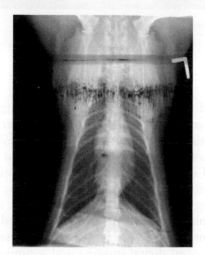

Figure 5.11. Dirty entrance rollers.

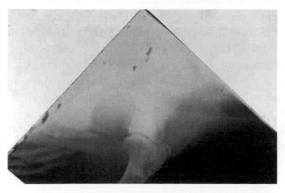

Figure 5.12. Dichroic stain. Image courtesy of Jeryl C. Jones, DVM.

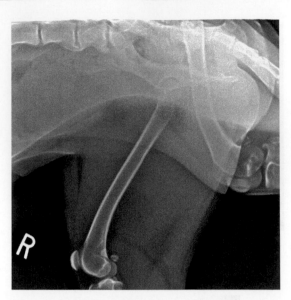

Figure 5.13.   Quantum mottle in pelvic and acetabular area.

more commonly seen artifacts are fogging, quantum mottle or noise, and nonparallel collimation.

Scatter radiation is one of the principal factors contributing to decreased film quality, causing a generalized fog that covers film and decreases contrast. In DR, fogging is due to imaging detectors being much more sensitive than film to scatter and background radiation. Factors contributing to fogging are high kVp, no grid or inadequate grid efficiency, inadequate collimation, and increased part size or tissue density. Fogging has an overall gray grainy appearance. Correct by using the technique chart, adding a grid when necessary and collimating. Fogging can be caused by faulty cassette light leak, placing a loaded film cassette in the radiographic room where it may be exposed, or a darkroom light leak.

Quantum mottle or quantum noise is caused by inadequate exposure. This artifact occurs both with film-screen and digital imaging and a similar appearance is produced. When mAs is deficient, the phrase "starving the detector" is frequently used to describe the lack of sufficient phosphor stimulation in DR. Correct by increasing mAs (and sometimes adjusting the kVp). Use a technique chart, collimate, but also remember to take into consideration the patient's physical condition. The same principle applies to film-screen systems. Quantum mottle is still due to inadequate mAS and it is more critical to adjust kVp as well as increase mAs (Fig. 5.13).

Nonparallel collimation is an artifact caused by not centering the anatomic region of interest to the middle of the DR panel. In DR, collimation edges must be parallel to the sides of the imaging plate or array or there is a noticeable loss of resolution. It occurs most frequently if the x-ray tube isn't centered to the DR panel or if the anatomic region of interest is offset on the panel. Correct by checking to ensure the tube is centered to the array and the anatomic part of interest is also centered on the DR panel/array, and collimate.

Positioning Aids and Alternative Restraint

Use of positioning aids and devices such as Head Ends, sandbags, foam wedges and blocks, head cradle positioning foam, compression restraint bands, masking tape, gauze rolls, and radiolucent gauze sponges is useful because they decrease the need for manual restraint, reduce repeat exposures to correct poor positioning, and reduce radiation exposure to the patient and holders (Fig. 6.1).

Safe Use of Restraint Devices

Caution must be used when utilizing these devices because they can harm the patient if not used properly. Never leave a sedated restrained animal unattended. Never place a sandbag over an animal's neck without dividing the sand to each side of the animal's neck (Fig. 6.2).

The full weight should never be on sensitive areas like an airway. Using foam positioning wedges will allow a patient to be easily placed in a true lateral position, keeping the gloved hands of the holders farther away from the area being imaged, and also will allow a quicker transition between anatomic regions. If imaging the thorax and abdomen on a large canine, the operator will be able to take the lateral thorax and the lateral cranial and caudal abdomen as quickly as it takes to change the film cassette, adjust technique, or choose the correct algorithm on the digital system. The whole patient is positioned, which makes it much less stressful on the patient, particularly if the patient is in pain. If your practice does a lot of orthopedic imaging, investing in a radiolucent table pad should be a consideration. Patients are more comfortable and easier to restrain as well as less sensitive to the noise from placing cassettes in the Bucky tray (Fig. 6.3).

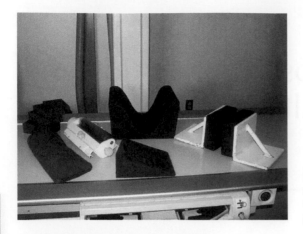

Figure 6.1. Positioning aids. *Clockwise from left,* sandbag, radiolucent positioning foam blocks, compression band, foam head cradle, Head End patient immobilization device, and foam wedge.

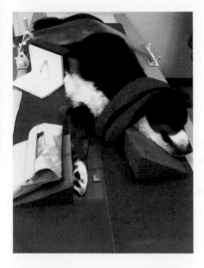

Figure 6.2. "Kona" is being restrained with a compression band over the abdomen. A Head End patient immobilization device is holding the right foreleg caudally so the left carpus can be imaged. A sandbag is placed over the neck with the sand divided so there is no heavy pressure on the neck. The positioning wedge is supporting the head, keeping it out of the field of view. A second positioning wedge is being used to hold the left carpus in position with another sandbag providing the weight needed to keep the wedge in place. Image courtesy of A. Reid Tyson, DVM.

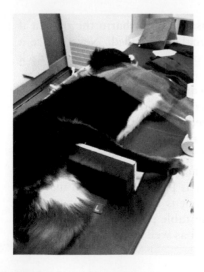

Figure 6.3. "Kona" is being restrained with the compression band over the shoulders. A Head End patient immobilization device is placed cranially to the left stifle with the right hind leg pulled cranially and propped on the immobilization device. Image courtesy of A. Reid Tyson, DVM.

Sedated Patient Restraint

Some restraint techniques are the result of technician ingenuity. For example, a large sedated dog is placed in a left lateral recumbent position and restrained with a compression band over the abdomen. A Head End patient immobilization device is holding the right foreleg caudally so left metacarpus and phalanges can be imaged. A sandbag is placed over the neck with the sand divided so there is no heavy pressure on the neck. The positioning wedge is supporting the head, keeping it out of the field of view. A second positioning wedge is being used to hold the left carpus in position, with another sandbag providing the weight needed to keep the wedge in place. The foot is oblique to separate the toes with tape and a radiolucent paddle was placed over the foot to keep the toes spread open for the image. This whole process was accomplished in just a few minutes (Fig. 6.4).

The technician then finalizes positioning and makes the exposure.

For the most secure restraint and to not affect respirations, a compression or restraint band should be applied across the shoulders if imaging the abdomen, pelvis, or a hind limb (Fig. 6.5).

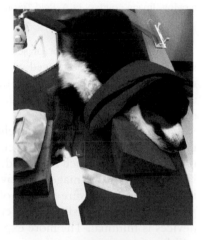

Figure 6.4. "Kona" is being restrained with a compression band over the abdomen. A Head End patient immobilization device is holding the right foreleg caudally so the left carpus can be imaged. A sandbag is placed over the neck with the sand divided so there is no heavy pressure on the neck. The positioning wedge is supporting the head, keeping it out of the field of view. A second positioning wedge is being used to hold the left forelimb in position, with another sandbag providing the weight needed to keep the wedge in place. A radiolucent paddle is placed over the foot to keep the toes spread open. Image courtesy of A. Reid Tyson, DVM.

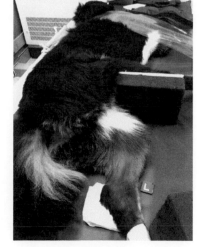

Figure 6.5. "Kona" is being restrained with the compression band over the shoulders. A Head End patient immobilization device is placed cranially to the left stifle with the right hind leg pulled cranially and propped on the immobilization device. The left tarsus is positioned for a lateral projection with gauze placed beneath the tarsal joint, and the second Head End patient immobilization device is used to keep the left hind limb in position. Image courtesy of A. Reid Tyson, DVM.

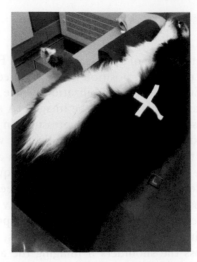

Figure 6.6.   A head cradle sponge is placed beneath the patient's head and the affected forelimb is pulled crani-ally and taped to the table. A compression band has been placed across the abdomen to keep "Kona" from moving. Image courtesy of A. Reid Tyson, DVM.

If imaging the shoulder or scapula, the compression band is placed over the pelvic area and the patient's head placed in a foam head cradle designed for positioning the head and neck. Depending upon the area of interest, one or both forelimbs can be pulled cranially and taped to the end of the table. Positioning the patient in an oblique position is safe and efficient (Fig. 6.6).

The first step is the tech or clinician must learn how each positioning aid should be used. There is a slight learning curve, but after practice, the process is more efficient and the positioning is much improved, creating a more diagnostic image to allow the veterinar-ian to interpret the images to provide better care for the patient and fewer retakes, thereby less radiation exposure to the holders and the patient. The cost to purchase a couple of positioning foam wedges, head cradle, and Head Ends or similar patient immobilization devices is minimal. The more expensive items, like the Head Ends and compression band, will last for many years if properly maintained and stored.

Radiation Safety

Health Physics

Following Wilhelm Conrad Roentgen's discovery of x-rays in 1895, Clarence Dally, an electrical engineer, and his brother, Charles, worked on the development of Thomas Edison's x-ray focus tube, or fluoroscope. Clarence was Mr. Edison's chief assistant during the experimental work. The Edison fluoroscope produced sharper images than Roentgen's fluoroscope, but Mr. Edison noted how "the x-ray had affected poisonously my assistant, Mr. Dally."[22] Clarence Dally started experiencing health issues shortly after first experimenting with x-rays. He eventually had both arms amputated due to carcinoma and was diagnosed with mediastinal cancer. He died a painful and horrific death at age 39 in 1904. He was the first American fatality from radiation exposure. Mr. Edison halted further x-ray tube development at his facilities and refused to be x-rayed for the rest of his 84 years. In 1903, as Mr. Dally was battling for his life, Mr. Edison was quoted as saying, "Don't talk to me about x-rays, I am afraid of them."[22]

In 1931, the first dose-limiting recommendations were made to protect radiation workers and the public. The practice of health physics is to provide radiation protection for workers and the public. Now, the National Council on Radiation Protection and Measurements (**NCRP**) reviews and revises recommended dose limits (**DL**). It is important to remember dose limits are for occupational exposure and do not include personal medical imaging procedures[2,23] (Table 7.1).

Radiologic Units

In 1981, the International Commission on Radiologic Units (**ICRU**) issued standards that were initially adopted everywhere except by the United States. The International System

Table 7.1. National Council on Radiation Protection and Measurements (NCRP) dose limit recommendations.[2,23]

Occupational Exposures

Effective dose: Annual 50 mSv (5,000 mrem)

Cumulative: 10 mSv × age (1,000 mrem × age)

Equivalent annual dose for tissues & organs

   Lens of eye: 150 mSv (15 rem)

   Skin, hands, feet: 500 mSv (50 rem)

Annual Public Exposures

Effective dose for frequent exposure: 1 mSv (100 mrem)

Effective dose for infrequent exposure: 5 mSv (500 mrem)

Equivalent dose for tissues and organs

   Lens of eye: 15 mSv (1,500 mrem)

   Skin, hands, feet: 50 mSv (5,000 mrem)

Annual Exposures—Children under 18 Years of Age

Effective dose: 1 mSv (100 mrem)

Equivalent dose for tissues & organs

   Lens of eye: 15 mSv (1,500 mrem)

   Skin, hands, feet: 50 mSv (5,000 mrem)

Embryo-Fetus Exposures

Total effective dose: 5 mSv (500 mrem)

Effective monthly dose: 0.5 mSv (50 mrem)

Annual Negligible Individual Dose: 0.01 mSv (10 mrem)

of Units (**SI**) is now used in the United States, but older terms are also still seen[2,23] (Tables 7.2 and 7.3).

Consistently adhering to established radiation safety practices is extremely important when using either film-screen or DR imaging systems. With DR imaging, it takes 10–30% more radiation exposure to produce a single DR image than a conventional radiographic exposure. The up side for DR is repeat exposures due to technique error or the need to see both bone and soft tissue is eliminated.

Safe operating procedures for a veterinary facility should include a good technique chart, positioning aids, protective lead apparel, and personnel monitoring dosimetry devices (Figs. 7.1 through 7.3).

All radiographic equipment must meet state regulation requirements. There should be at least two pairs of flexible lead gloves and aprons in good condition available for use in restraining a patient for imaging (Fig. 7.4).

Thyroid shields are not required but are recommended, particularly if the practice has a fluoroscopic unit in use. If using DR, though it may be easier to overexpose and correct with the workstation, it will affect image quality and violate the ALARA concept.

Table 7.2. Radiologic units and definition of terms.[2,23]

Absorbed dose: The energy imparted to matter by ionizing radiation per unit mass of irradiated material at the place of interest. The unit is the gray (Gy), defined to be an energy absorption of 1 J/kg. The older term used was the rad, defined to be energy absorption of 100 ergs per gram.[23]

Activity: Radioactivity. The becquerel (Bq) is the unit of activity. 1 Gbq = 3.7×10^{10} Bq = 1 Ci.[23]

Becquerel (Bq): Special name for the SI units of radioactivity. One becquerel is equal to disintegration per second.[2,23]

Dose equivalent: Radiation quantity used in radiation protection that expresses the dose on a common scale for all radiations. The unit of equivalent dose is the sievert (Sv) or rem.[2,23]

Exposure: The measure of the ionization produced in air by gamma rays or x-rays. The quantity of radiation intensity is expressed in air kerma (Gy), roentgen (R), or Coulombs per kilogram (C/kg.)[2]

Gray (Gy): Special name for the SI unit of absorbed dose and air kerma. 1 Gy = 1 J/kg = 100 rad.[23]

Negligible individual dose: Level of effective dose that is considered insignificant so further efforts to improve radiation protection aren't justified. The recommended negligible individual dose is 0.01 mSv/y.[23]

rad (radiation absorbed dose): Old term for special unit for absorbed dose, kerma, and specific energy imparted. 1 rad is 0.01 J absorbed per kilogram of any material. It is also defined as 100 ergs per gram. The term has been replaced by gray. 1 rad = 0.01 Gy.[2]

rem (radiation equivalent man): The special unit for dose equivalent and effective dose. It has been replaced by the sievert (Sv) in the SI system. 1 rem = 0.01 Sv.[2]

sievert (Sv): The unit of equivalent dose or effective dose in the SI system. 1 Sv = 1 J/kg^{-1} = 100 rem.[2]

Table 7.3. Radiologic unit and SI unit conversion table.[2,23]

Quantity	Customary Unit			SI Unit	
	Name		Symbol	Name	Symbol
Exposure	roentgen		R	air kerma	Gy_a
Absorbed dose	rad		rad	gray	Gy_1
Effective dose	rem		rem	sievert	Sv
Radioactivity	curie		Ci	Becquerel	Bq
Multiply	R	by	0.01	to obtain	Gy_a
Multiply	rad	by	0.01	to obtain	Gy_t
Multiply	rem	by	0.01	to obtain	Sv
Multiply	Ci	by	3.7×10^{10}	to obtain	Bq
Multiply	R	by	2.58×10^{-4}	to obtain	C/kg

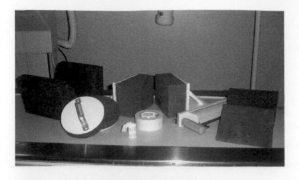

Figure 7.1. Positioning and restraint aids.

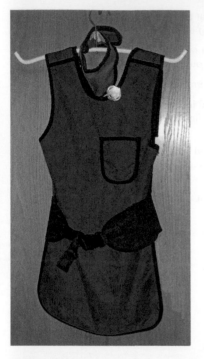

Figure 7.2. Wide belt lead apron with thyroid shield and radiation dosimetry badge on collar of lead apron.

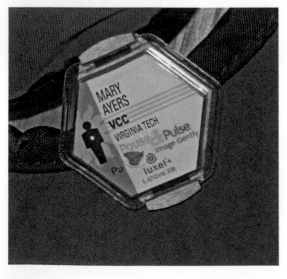

Figure 7.3. Radiation dosimetry badge.

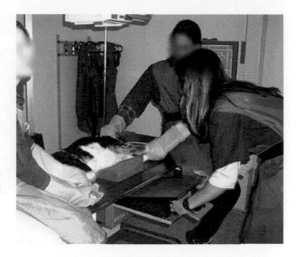

Figure 7.4. Imaging of a nonsedated patient. The personnel restraining the patient are wearing appropriate lead apparel. The person who is positioning does not need to wear lead apparel. Foam wedge is being used to position the patient in lateral recumbency.

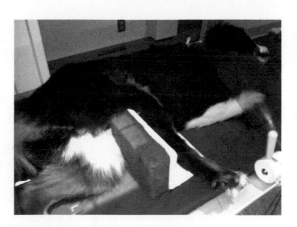

Figure 7.5. Alternative restraint technique being used on a lightly sedated patient.

CHAPTER 7

ALARA Concept

The **ALARA** concept simply means radiation exposure in the workplace should be **As Low As Reasonably Achievable**. To practice the ALARA concept, you should develop and use a technique chart; become proficient in patient positioning; wear appropriate lead apparel; use chemical restraint when possible; and consistently use positioning aids like restraint bands, sandbags, tape, foam wedges and blocks, and Head End patient immobilization devices (Fig. 7.5).

Each small animal practice should have lead aprons and gloves or mittens that are 0.5 mm thick lead equivalent, and the apparel should fit well and be used (Figs. 7.6 and 7.7).

Thyroid shields are also recommended, particularly if a limited number of staff provide manual restraint of patients during imaging.

In most states, manual restraint of patients is a common practice, so there is concern about the results of long-term cumulative exposure to radiation. It is the responsibility of the veterinary practitioner and staff to do everything possible to keep radiation exposure

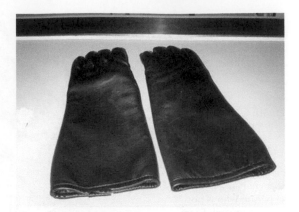

Figure 7.6.   Pair of flexible lead gloves.

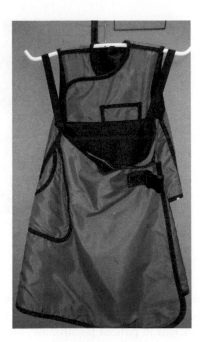

Figure 7.7.   Lead vest and apron.

in the practice as low as reasonably possible. The same person should not consistently hold every patient for imaging. Minimize personnel in the radiographic room during imaging and rotate personnel if possible to decrease occupational radiation exposure. Wear a radiation dosimetry badge outside of the lead apron on a collar to keep an accurate record of exposure. Change the radiation dosimetry badges at least quarterly. Inspect lead gloves at least monthly for cracks or tears in the lead (Fig. 7.8).

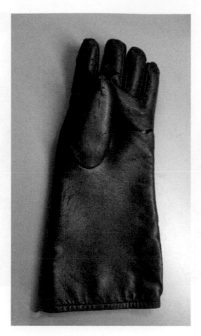

Figure 7.8. Lead glove with tear on palmar side of glove.

Maximize shielding between personnel and the x-ray tube by making exposures from outside of the room or behind a protective lead equivalent barrier. Pregnant workers should declare their pregnancy to their supervisor as soon as possible so special considerations can be applied. Pregnant staff should not restrain patients for imaging. They should not be in the radiographic room at all during the first trimester, when an exposure is being made. A second radiation dosimetry badge should be ordered for the pregnant staff worker and be worn at waist level. The most hazardous period for the fetus in regard to radiation exposure is from week 2 through week 10. During this time, the fetus's major organ systems are developing. The dose limit for the fetus for the entire pregnancy is 5 mSv/9 months (500 mrem/9 months).

An example of poor radiation safety practices is visiting a small animal practice and finding lead gloves so old and stiff that the holder could not possibly hold a patient or get his or her hands inside the gloves. At least one lead apron is present but radiation dosimetry badges are often not worn, just stored outside of the radiographic room, sometimes in a desk drawer. The badge reports will look great for an official state inspection since they are minimal and there is no way an inspector would know unless it is a surprise inspection and a patient is being imaged when the inspector walks in. Since a pair of lead gloves and a lead apron are hung in the room, and the practice has the state-required postings and x-ray tube inspection report, the state regulations have been met. Rarely are positioning aids seen in the radiographic room. The techs will state something was mentioned about positioning aids in school but they have found it is easier to just hold the patient, not realizing the image quality is deficient because their positioning skills are deficient. When films are sent to a referral practice and the veterinary radiologist reviews

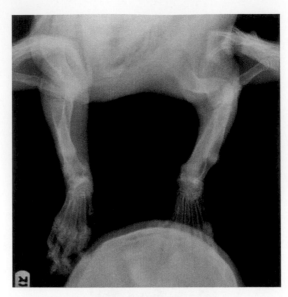

Figure 7.9.   Holder's hands and head in the primary beam.

the images, the radiologist can also evaluate the joints in the holder's fingers because sometimes the holder's hands and wrists will be seen holding. What is that unusual artifact? It is the rims of the holder's glasses in the primary beam because the view was not collimated and the holder did not wear appropriate lead apparel. Does this scenario seem outrageous? It shouldn't, because all of the incidents mentioned in this scenario are real. The author combined the different incidents to form one scenario, but all have occurred. Remember certain cells and organs within the body are more sensitive to radiation, including gonads, lenses of the eyes, GI tract, and thyroid gland (Fig. 7.9).

Section 2

Radiographic Positioning

General Principles and Terminology

Pets are such an integral part of the family that when they become ill or injured, the veterinary client expects the best quality care be given, particularly due to the advancements in technology and medicine. Part of providing quality care is accurately diagnosing and treating the patient using diagnostic tools such as radiographic imaging. The veterinary technician's role in this process has grown from providing wide-range nursing care, anesthesia support duties, and laboratory tasks to performing basic to more advanced radiographic imaging. It is important for the technician to understand the positional terminology, learn how to position the patient for a variety of imaging studies, and incorporate the use of positioning aids to accurately and efficiently attain the images while following radiation safety practices. Technicians must also learn to review their images to evaluate for positioning technique and technical quality and to be able to correct errors. The first steps to becoming proficient in radiography are learning basic positioning views, correct positional terminology, required patient preparation, and methods of restraint. Good positioning skills are mandatory to become a successful radiographer.

Positioning Terminology

The direction the x-ray beam travels through the body of the patient designates the view taken. Ventrodorsal (VD) indicates the patient is lying in a dorsal recumbent position and the x-ray beam is entering the patient ventrally and is exiting through the back of the patient. If the patient is lying in a sternal recumbent position, the x-ray beam is entering the body through the back and exits ventrally. Dorsopalmar and dorsoplantar are the terms used when the x-ray beam enters the front and exits through the back of the distal portion of the carpal and tarsal joints and below, respectively. For the proximal extremities, craniocaudal is the term used when the x-ray beam enters the front and exits the back of an extremity. Caudocranial is used when the x-ray beam enters through the back of an extremity and exits through the front[15] (Table 8.1).

Right and left anatomic lead equivalent markers should be used to designate the right or left side of the body or to identify an extremity. For a lateral view of the pelvis or spine the lead marker should be placed dorsal to the spine or pelvis within the collimated area but not in the anatomy and not ventrally. For a lateral view of the thorax or abdomen, the right or left marker should be placed ventrally, within the collimated field but not in the anatomy and not dorsally. An example is to place the left marker in the

Table 8.1.   Positioning terminology.

Term	Definition
Caudal	Refers to parts of the head, neck, or trunk facing toward the hind part of the body from any set point. Also refers to those aspects of the limbs above the carpal and tarsal joints facing in the direction of the hind part of the body
Cranial	Refers to parts of the neck, trunk, and tail facing the direction of the head from any set point. Also refers to superior or anterior aspect of a body part or limb above the carpal and tarsal joints
Distal	Refers to any part away from the center of the body
Dorsal	Refers to the back or posterior part of the body; opposite of ventral
Lateral	X-ray beam enters either the right or left side of the body and exits on the opposite side
Mediolateral	X-ray beam enters the limb medially and exits laterally
Palmar	Refers to the posterior or inferior aspect of the forelimb from the carpus, distally
Plantar	Refers to the posterior or inferior aspect of the hind limb from the tarsus, distally
Proximal	Refers to the end of a limb or other part closest to the point of attachment
Recumbent	Refers to the animal lying down
Rostral	Toward the head or nares
Superior and inferior	Refers to the upper and lower dental arcades, respectively
Ventral	Refers to the abdominal or sternal surface of the body

axillary region when doing a lateral thorax. The marker is in the collimated field but not in the anatomy. For ventrodorsal or dorsoventral views, the left or right is placed lateral to the body within the collimated field but not in the anatomy. When doing a dorsopalmar view of the carpus, the right or left marker should be placed lateral to the joint (Fig. 8.1)

When doing a lateral or lateral oblique view of an extremity, the marker should be placed cranially within the collimated field but not in the anatomic region being imaged (Fig. 8.2 and Table 8.2).

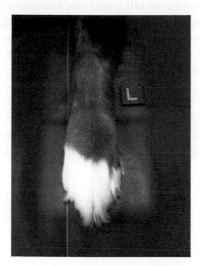

Figure 8.1. Correct anatomic marker placement for dorsopalmar projection of the left metacarpus.

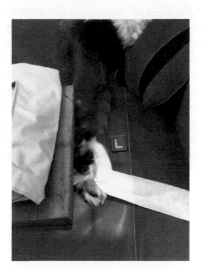

Figure 8.2. Correct anatomic marker placement for lateral oblique projection of the left metacarpus.

CHAPTER 8

Table 8.2. Positioning term abbreviations.

Term	Abbreviation
Left	(L)
Right	(R)
Dorsal	(D)
Ventral	(V)
Oblique	(O)
Fore	(F)
Hind	(H)
Cranial	(Cr)
Caudal	(Cd)
Palmar	(Pa)
Plantar	(Pl)
Ventrodorsal	(VD)
Dorsoventral	(DV)

Room Setup

Before the patient is brought into the room, the technician will need to prepare the room for the study. The supplies needed are the anatomic markers, caliper for measuring the patient, technique chart on the correct page, and the correct size film- screen cassettes; the darkroom needs to be prepared to process the image and properly label the film with patient information or enter information into the computer for digital imaging, a technique sheet to record kVp and mAs with the routine views normally requested for the exam needs to be prepared, and the positioning aids to use need to be chosen. Remember to center the part of interest to the center of the film cassette or DR panel and collimate. For extremity work and headwork, use the small focal spot for anatomic parts measuring 10 cm or less to improve the quality of the image. Measure the patient after placement in the recumbent position, not standing on the table. If assistance is needed in imaging the patient, ask for help before the patient is on the table.

Align the x-ray tube to the Bucky tray containing the film cassette or the DR panel. The source-image distance (SID) should be minimally 40 inches for a 300 mA generator. If the x-ray generator is more powerful, like a 400–600 mA generator, the SID can be increased to 44 inches if recommended by the equipment manufacturer. Being consistent is important because there is a difference in heart size when imaging a thorax at 40 inches versus 44 inches.

Patient Preparation

The patient's coat should be dry and debris-free. Wet hair and debris create artifacts on the radiographic image and may hinder the veterinarian in interpreting the image. Iodine-based skin medications are radiopaque and should be removed, if possible, as well as bandages and splints. Depending upon the anatomic region being imaged, collars and harnesses should be removed. If the abdomen is the area of interest, enemas or fasting may be called for.

It is preferred to use chemical restraint with positioning aids to image the small animal patient. In some states, manually restraining a patient is against state regulations. The goal is to minimize radiation exposure and attain quality imaging. If it is necessary to manually restrain a patient because chemical restraint is contraindicated, strictly adhere to radiation safety practices. The holder(s) should wear lead aprons and gloves while restraining the patient and also use positioning aids to minimize the number of people in the room. Collimate to the anatomic region of interest, and stand as far away from the primary beam as possible. Lead aprons and gloves are designed to protect the holder from scatter radia-tion so do not place gloved hands in the primary beam. A compression band is an excellent positioning aid to use to securely hold one end of the patient on the table when imaging an anatomic region cranially or caudally to the band.

Remember that animals not sedated for imaging studies are not very tolerant and need the technician to speak softly and consolingly to them, position well and quickly, and be cognizant of any change in the patient's behavior. Most likely the patient will be in pain and anxious, thereby unpredictable in regard to behavior. Loud noises and hurried movements can be alarming to a pet. This is particularly important if the animal is seriously injured. The ideal image may not be attainable, but diagnostic images are generally possible. It may be necessary to take horizontal beam projections if the patient cannot be turned due to a suspected fractured spine. This is the type of imaging challenge where the technician has to be innovative (Figs. 8.3 through 8.6).

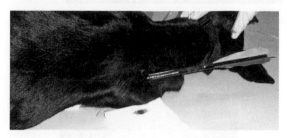

Figure 8.3.   Canine patient impaled by an arrow.

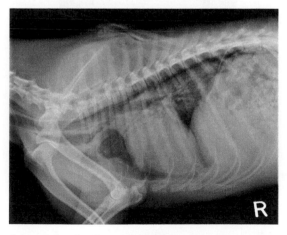

Figure 8.4.   Lateral view of thorax showing the arrow's path.

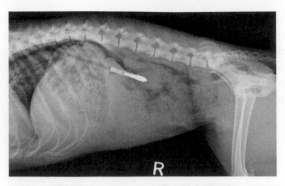

Figure 8.5.   Lateral view of the abdomen with arrow's tip.

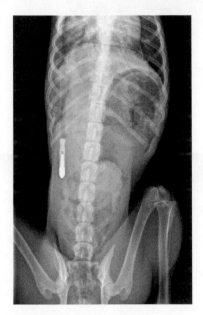

Figure 8.6.   VD abdomen with arrow's tip.

Horizontal Beam Views

Horizontal beam views are views taken with the patient in lateral, dorsal, or ventral recumbent positions or with the patient standing in lateral, dorsal, or ventral standing positions. Horizontal beam views called lateral decubitus views can be used for visualization of free air in the abdomen and pleural effusion in the thorax. Horizontal beam views for mediastinal masses are taken with the patient held upright in a VD position. They are also used for imaging trauma patients when spinal fractures are suspected or even fractures of the extremities. If a practice has a permanently mounted DR panel in the table, horizontal beam imaging is not possible. If the DR panel is tethered so it can be removed from the table, it is important to remember the area of interest must be centered to the DR panel and not offset to one side or the other. When a horizontal beam view is requested, it is important to have the clinician clarify the projection needed (Figs. 8.7 through 8.10).

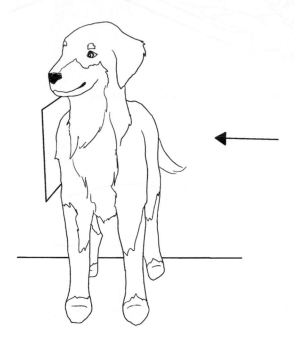

Figure 8.7. Horizontal beam standing lateral projection.

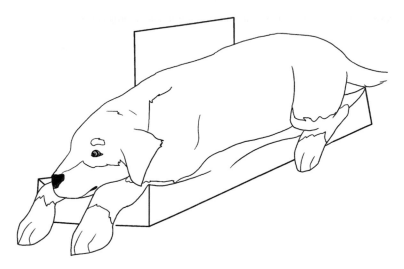

Figure 8.8. Horizontal beam recumbent lateral projection.

CHAPTER 8

of the extremity, with a particular portion nearest the DR panel. In the table, however, it is not always possible. If the DR panel is required to be in the table, it is not always possible to use the area of the panel not to be centered to the DR panel and not cover to another extremity. When a horizontal beam view is required, it is important to have the clinical view the principles of positioning, see Figs. 8.7 through 8.10.

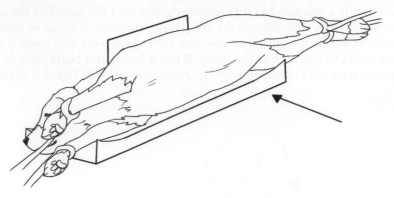

Figure 8.9.   Horizontal beam recumbent lateral position for VD view.

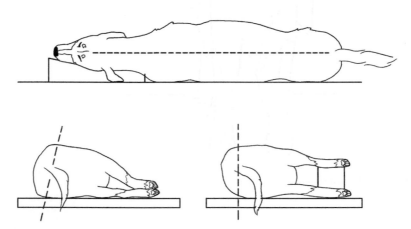

Figure 8.10.   Positioning diagram illustrating a patient in a true lateral projection.

Small Animal Positioning—Forelimb

9

Scapula

The routine views of the scapula are lateral and caudocranial views. Please note two lateral views may need to be taken to completely visualize the scapula, one for the body of the scapula and a second view for the neck of the scapula.

Sedation: Recommended.

View: Lateral View to Visualize the Body of the Scapula

Center and Measurement Point: Mid-body of the scapula.
Manual restraint required for this view. Place the patient in a lateral recumbent position, affected side down. Grasp the down leg below the elbow, extending the elbow joint so it cannot bend, and push dorsally, forcing the body of the scapula dorsally so it is seen bulging above the dorsal spinous processes of the thoracic vertebra. At the same time, grasp the up leg and pull ventrally and caudally, which will rotate the thorax slightly, and further isolate the scapular body (Figs. 9.1 and 9.2).

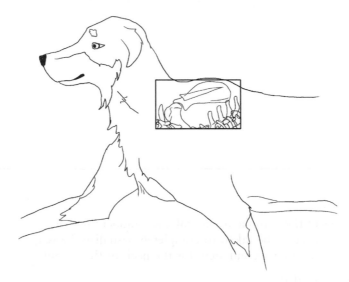

Figure 9.1.   Lateral view scapular body illustration.

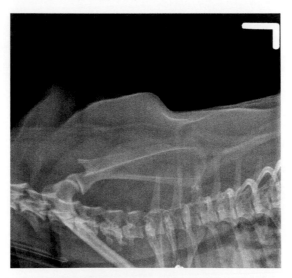

Figure 9.2.   Lateral view scapular body.

View: Lateral View to Visualize the Scapular Neck

Center and Measurement Point: Scapular neck.
Manual restraint required for this view. Place the patient in a lateral recumbent position, affected side down. Pull affected limb cranially and ventrally while pulling the unaffected leg caudally to visualize the scapular neck (Figs. 9.3 and 9.4).

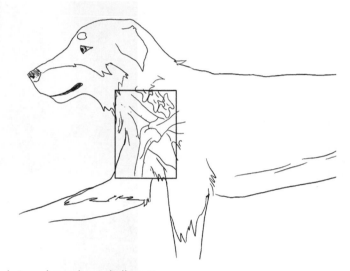

Figure 9.3. Lateral view of scapular neck illustration.

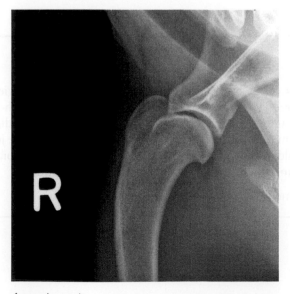

Figure 9.4. Lateral view of scapular neck.

View: Caudocranial View

Center and Measurement Point: Mid-body of the scapula.

Place the patient in a dorsal recumbent position with the forelegs extended cranially. Rotate the patient's sternum away from the affected side, approximately 10 degrees, to remove the ribs from the proximity of the body of the scapula (Figs. 9.5 and 9.6).

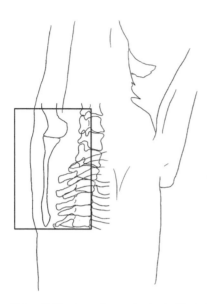

Figure 9.5.   CdCr view of scapular body illustration.

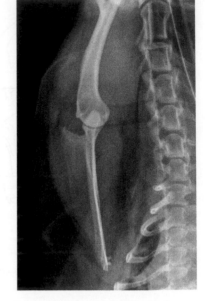

Figure 9.6.   CdCr view of scapular body.

Shoulder

The routine views of the shoulder are lateral and craniocaudal views. The lateral shoulder view is frequently used to confirm the presence of osteochondrosis lesions, normally located on the caudal aspect of the humeral head near midline. The trachea and the manubrium of the sternum must be moved away from the joint to properly visualize the shoulder joint. An additional view to visualize the bicipital groove is helpful in evaluating the supraspinatus tendon for calcifications.

Sedation: Recommended.

View: Lateral View

Center and Measurement Point: Shoulder joint.

Place the patient in a lateral recumbent position, affected side down. Pull affected limb cranially and ventrally while pulling the unaffected leg caudally. Slightly extend the patients head and neck dorsally to remove the trachea from over the joint. The joint can be palpated by running fingers up the cranial surface of the humerus to the joint (Figs. 9.7 and 9.8).

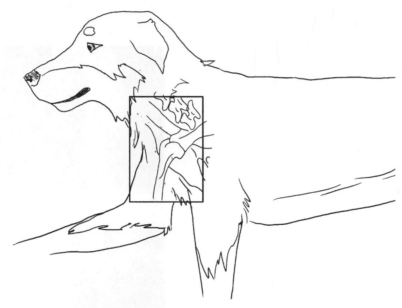

Figure 9.7.   Lateral view illustration.

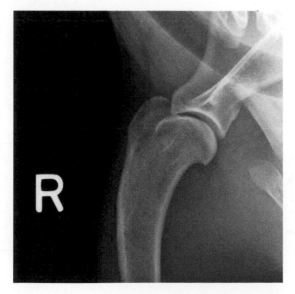

Figure 9.8.   Lateral view.

View: Caudocranial View

Center and Measurement Point: Shoulder joint.

Place the patient in a dorsal recumbent position with the forelegs extended cranially. To avoid an oblique projection of the shoulder joint, do not rotate the humerus (Figs. 9.9 through 9.11).

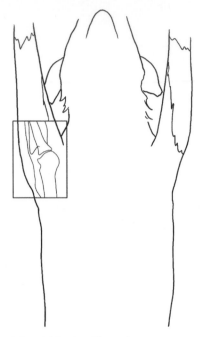

Figure 9.9.   CdCr view illustration.

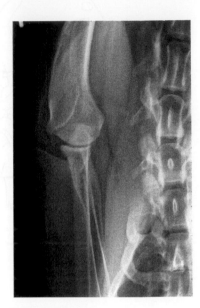

Figure 9.11.   CdCr view.

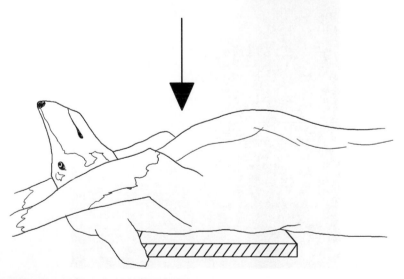

Figure 9.10.   CdCr view, side projection illustration.

Bicipital Groove

Center and Measurement Point: Head of the humerus.

Film-Screen Cassette: Place the patient in a sternal recumbent position with the head turned slightly away from the affected shoulder without rotating the thorax. The thorax must remain upright. The elbow joint of the affected leg should be flexed so the shoulder joint is projected over the proximal third of the radius and ulna. The film-screen cassette is placed in the crook of elbow joint. Palpate the head of the humerus to find the bicipital groove and center the collimator light over that point. Collimate tightly to the area of interest; the x-ray beam is projected through the bicipital groove (Figs. 9.12 and 9.13).

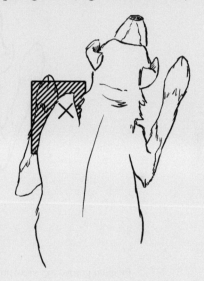

Figure 9.12.   Bicipital groove top view projection illustration with film cassette.

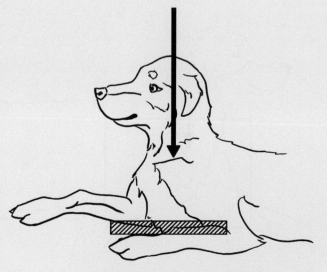

Figure 9.13.   Bicipital groove side view projection illustration with film cassette.

Continued

DR Panel: Place the patient in a sternal recumbent position with the head turned slightly away from the affected shoulder without rotating the thorax. The thorax must remain upright. The elbow joint of the affected leg should be flexed so the shoulder joint is projected over the proximal third of the radius and ulna. Palpate the head of the humerus to find the bicipital groove and center the collimator light over that point. Collimate tightly to the area of interest. Without moving the shoulder, humerus, or elbow, gently move the radius and ulna slightly lateral to allow the bicipital groove to be projected onto the DR panel (Figs. 9.14 through 9.16).

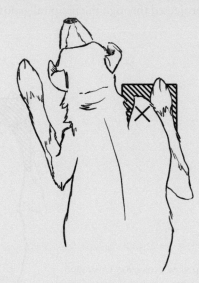

Figure 9.14. Bicipital groove top view projection illustration with DR panel.

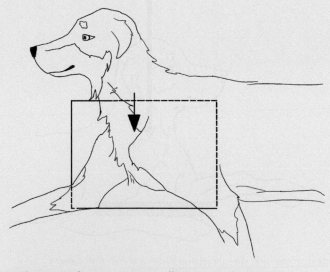

Figure 9.15. Bicipital groove side view projection illustration with DR panel.

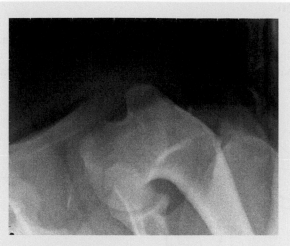

Figure 9.16.   Bicipital groove image.

Humerus

The routine views of the humerus are lateral, caudocranial, or craniocaudal views. The craniocaudal view is generally used when the patient is unable to extend forelimb cranially due to pain or fracture.

Sedation: Recommended.

Centering Point: Mid-shaft of the humerus.

Measurement Point: Shoulder joint.

View: Lateral View

Place the patient in a lateral recumbent position, affected side down. Pull affected limb cranially and ventrally while pulling the unaffected leg caudally, out of the field of view. Slightly extend the patient's head and neck dorsally to remove the trachea from over the head of the humerus (Figs. 9.17 and 9.18).

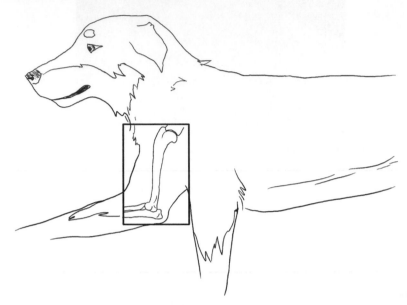

Figure 9.17.   Lateral view illustration.

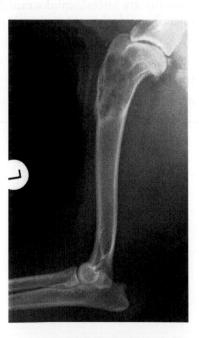

Figure 9.18.   Lateral view.

View: Caudocranial View

Place the patient in a dorsal recumbent position with the forelegs extended cranially. The affected leg should remain as parallel to the tabletop as possible to reduce distortion. Collimate to include the elbow and shoulder joints in the view (Figs. 9.19 and 9.20).

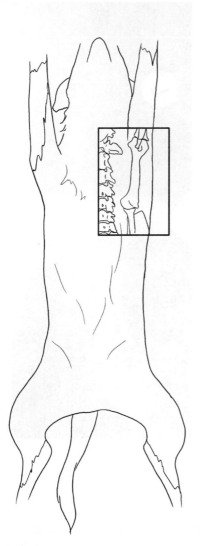

Figure 9.19.   CdCr view illustration.

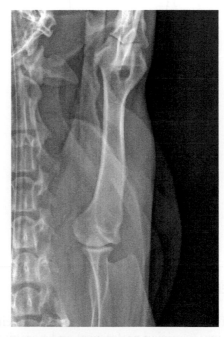

Figure 9.20.   CdCr view.

View: Craniocaudal View

Place the patient in a dorsal recumbent position with the affected limb extended caudally and the plane of the humerus parallel to the tabletop. The forelimb should be abducted slightly away from the thorax to prevent superimposition of the ribs over the humerus (Figs. 9.21 and 9.22).

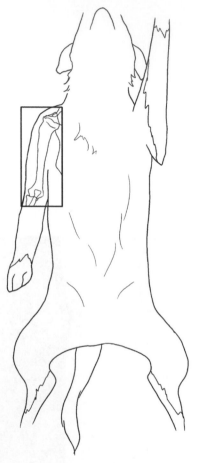

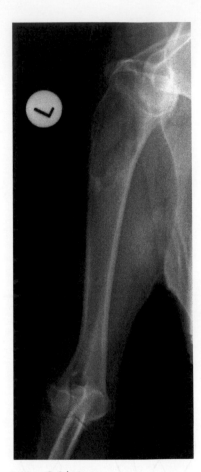

Figure 9.21.   CrCd view illustration.

Figure 9.22.   CrCd view.

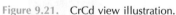

Elbow

The routine views of the elbow are either a 45-degree or 90-degree flexed lateral view (clinician preference) and a craniocaudal view. Supplementary views are hyperflexed lateral for evaluation of an ununited anconeal process and oblique views. OFA evaluation of the elbow joint only requires the hyperflexed lateral view.

Sedation: Recommended.

Center and Measurement Point: Humeroulnar joint.

View: Lateral View

Place the patient in a lateral recumbent position, affected side down. Position the affected field of view limb cranially and ventrally while pulling the unaffected leg caudally, out of the field of view. The degree of flexion is 45 degrees or 90 degrees, clinician preference (Figs. 9.23 and 9.24).

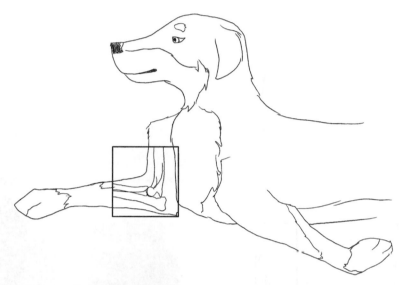

Figure 9.23.   Lateral view illustration 90 degrees.

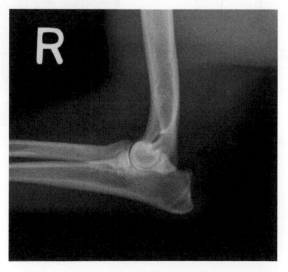

Figure 9.24.   Lateral view.

View: Craniocaudal View

Place the patient in a sternal recumbent position with the affected forelimb fully extended. The patient's head should be elevated and turned away from the affected side and the thorax should remain upright. The humerus, elbow joint, and radius and ulna should remain aligned to ensure a true CrCd view. If the elbow joint cannot be fully extended, the x-ray beam should be angled 10 to 20 degrees to open the joint to evaluate the radial joint surface[15] (Figs. 9.25 and 9.26).

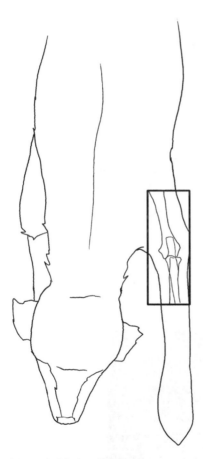

Figure 9.25.   CrCd view illustration.

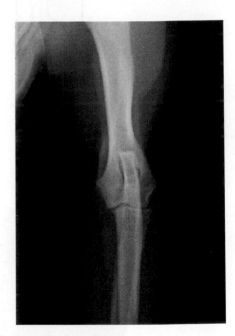

Figure 9.26.   CrCd view.

View: Supplementary Hyperflexed Lateral View

Place the patient in a lateral recumbent position, affected side down. Position the affected field of view limb cranially and ventrally while pulling the unaffected leg caudally, out of the field of view. Keeping the carpus in a true lateral position, move the carpus toward the neck to hyperflex the elbow joint. This will also keep the elbow joint in a true lateral position.

The hyperflexed lateral view is the only view required for an OFA evaluation (Figs. 9.27 and 9.28).

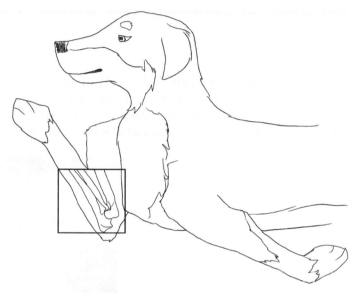

Figure 9.27.   Hyperflexed lateral view illustration.

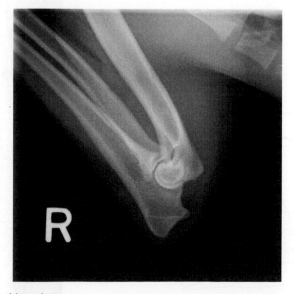

Figure 9.28.   Hyperflexed lateral view.

Radius and Ulna

The routine views of the radius and ulna are lateral and craniocaudal views.

Sedation: Recommended.

Center Point: Midpoint of the radius and ulna.

Measurement Point: Elbow joint.

View: Lateral View

Place the patient in a lateral recumbent position, affected side down. Slightly flex the elbow and pull the radius and ulna cranially away from the body and move the unaffected leg caudally, out of the field of view. The radius and ulna should be centered on the film cassette or DR panel. Collimate to include the elbow and carpal joints (Figs. 9.29 and 9.30).

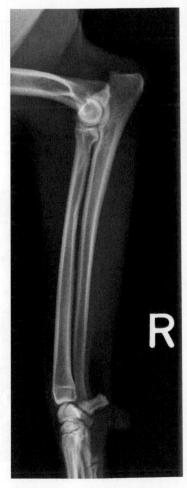

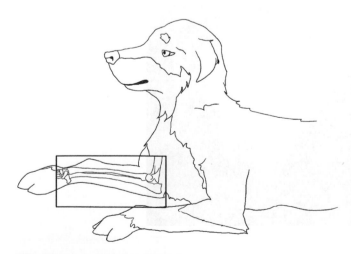

Figure 9.29.   Lateral view illustration.

Figure 9.30.   Lateral view.

View: Craniocaudal View

Place the patient in a sternal recumbent position with the affected forelimb fully extended. The patient's head should be elevated and turned away from the affected side and the thorax should remain upright. Center the radius and ulna to the film cassette or DR panel. Collimate to include the elbow and carpal joints (Figs. 9.31 and 9.32).

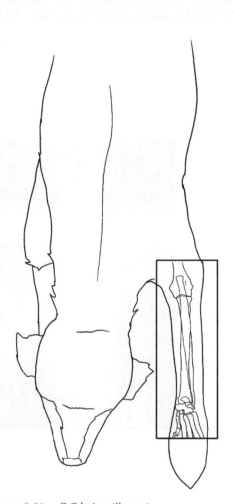

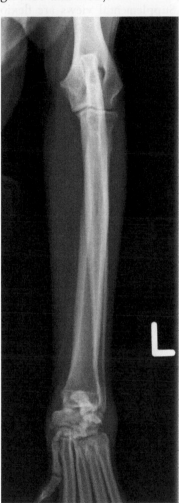

Figure 9.31.   CrCd view illustration.   Figure 9.32.   CrCd view.

Carpus

The routine views for the carpus are dorsopalmar (DPa) and lateral views. Supplemental views are flexion, extension, and oblique views.

Sedation: Recommended.

Center Point: Carpal joint.

Measurement Point: Carpal joint.

CHAPTER 9

View: Lateral View

Place the patient in a lateral recumbent position, affected side down. Slightly flex the elbow and pull the radius and ulna cranially away from the body and move the unaffected leg caudally, out of the field of view. The carpal joint should be centered on the film cassette or DR panel. Collimate to include the distal third of the radius and ulna and the metacarpal bones. Supplemental views are flexion, extension, and 45-degree oblique dorsopalmar-mediolateral and dorsopalmar-lateromedial views off the dorsopalmar view (Figs. 9.33 and 9.34).

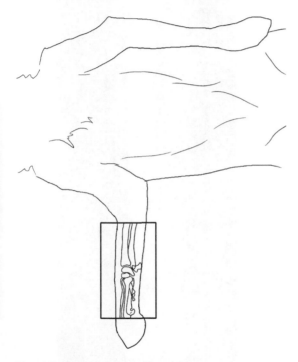

Figure 9.33.   Lateral view illustration.

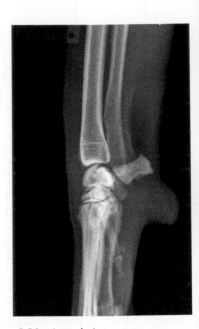

Figure 9.34.   Lateral view.

View: *Dorsopalmar View*

Place the patient in a sternal recumbent position with the affected forelimb fully extended. The patient's head should be elevated and turned away from the affected side and the thorax should remain upright. Center the carpal joint to the film cassette or DR panel. Collimate to include the distal third of the radius and ulna and the metacarpal bones (Figs. 9.35 and 9.36).

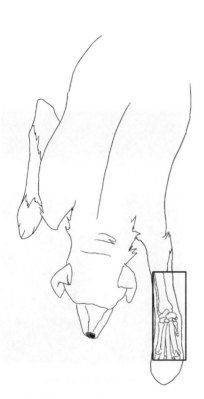

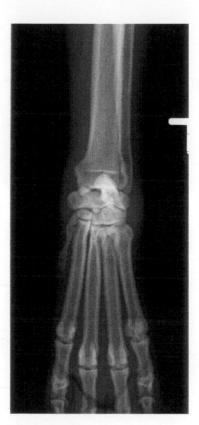

Figure 9.35.   DPa view illustration.

Figure 9.36.   DPa view.

CHAPTER 9

Supplemental Views: Flexion, Extension, Oblique, and Stress Views

For flexion and extension views, care should be taken to keep the joint in a true lateral projection. For oblique views, the carpal joint is rotated 45 degrees dorsopalmar view (Figs. 9.37 through 9.42).

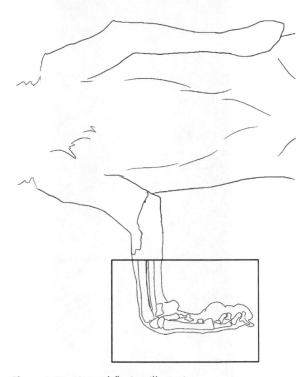

Figure 9.37.   Lateral flexion illustration.

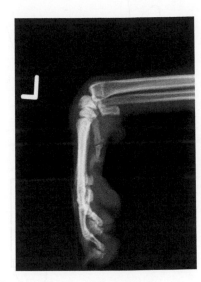

Figure 9.38.   Lateral flexion view.

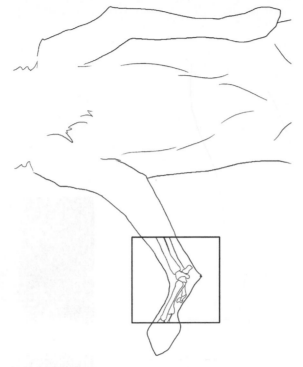

Figure 9.39. Lateral extension illustration.

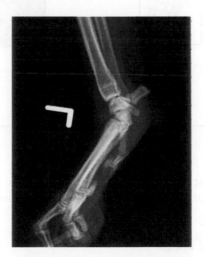

Figure 9.40. Lateral extension view.

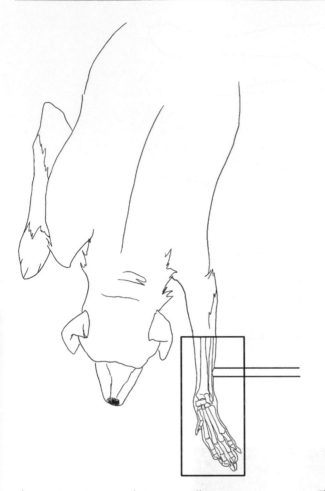
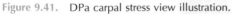

Figure 9.41.   DPa carpal stress view illustration.

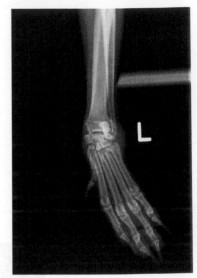

Figure 9.42.   DPa carpal stress view.

Metacarpus, Digits

The routine views for the metacarpus and phalanges are DPa and lateral views. Supplemental views are lateral views of the individual digits.

Sedation: Recommended.

Center Point: Metacarpal bones.

Measurement Point: Metacarpal bones.

View: Lateral View

Place the patient in a lateral recumbent position, affected side down. Slightly flex the elbow and pull the radius and ulna cranially away from the body and move the unaffected leg caudally, out of the field of view. The metacarpal bones and phalanges should be centered on the film cassette or DR panel. Collimate to include the carpal joint and the tips of the digits. Supplemental lateral view of the digits: Separating and taping the toes apart in a slightly oblique lateral view will separate the digits (Figs. 9.43 and 9.44).

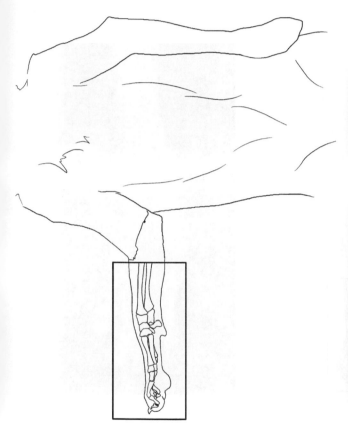

Figure 9.43.   Lateral view illustration.

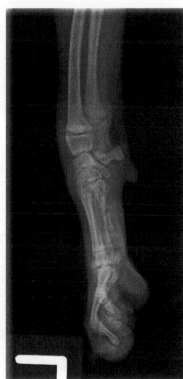

Figure 9.44.   Lateral view.

Dorsopalmar View

Place the patient in a sternal recumbent position with the affected forelimb fully extended. The patient's head should be elevated and turned away from the affected side and the thorax should remain upright. Center the metacarpal bones to the film cassette or DR panel. Collimate to include the distal third of the carpal joint and the tips of the digits. Sometimes it may be necessary to tape the foot flat to achieve a true DPa view of these bones (Figs. 9.45 and 9.46).

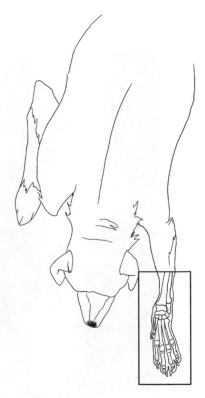

Figure 9.45.   DPa view illustration.

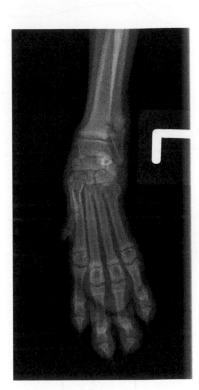

Figure 9.46.   DPa view.

Small Animal Positioning—Pelvis and Hind Limb

Pelvis

The routine views for pelvic imaging are extended leg ventrodorsal (VD) and lateral. Other views often requested are the VD frog-leg view and the acetabular rim view.

Sedation: Heavy sedation or general anesthesia.

Center Point: Greater trochanter.

Measurement Point: Greater trochanter.

View: Lateral View

For the lateral view of the pelvis, place the patient in a lateral recumbent position with the affected side down. Make sure the chest and abdomen are in a true lateral position, using positioning wedges beneath the sternum or cranial abdomen, as needed. The bottom femur should be in a neutral position, which means it is slightly pulled cranial with the stifle flexed, as if the patient were standing. The upper leg should be pulled caudally and either manually restrained or taped to the table. The tuber ischii should be superimposed. Sometimes a positioning wedge is needed between the hind legs for larger breed dogs (Figs. 10.1 and 10.2).

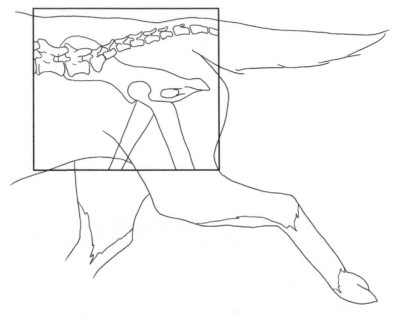

Figure 10.1.   Lateral view illustration.

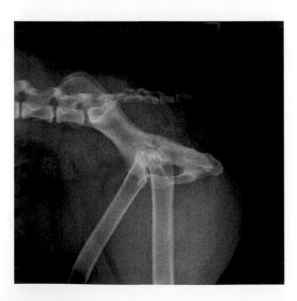

Figure 10.2.   Lateral view.

View: Ventrodorsal View Legs Extended

Place the patient in dorsal recumbent position with the head in a head cradle positioning sponge with the Head End against the shoulders. Make sure the sternum and spine are superimposed as you extend the hind legs. Grasp the tarsi, flex the stifles, and pull the tarsi toward you, making sure the patient's midline is centered to the table, and apply equal traction to each leg. The cranial border of the image is the crest of the ilium and the caudal border should include the stifle joints. The patellae are centered between the femoral condyles. For no sedation or lightly sedated patients, it may be necessary to have a holder at both ends of the patient to use traction to efficiently extend the lower legs to attain a properly positioned VD pelvis. If the patient is under heavy sedation, the technician can use a compression band with Head End and head cradle positioning foam to restrain the upper body so one holder can extend the lower legs. Depending upon the flexibility of the patient and the level of sedation, no holders may be necessary. Positioning may be possible by adding roll gauze or tape to keep the legs parallel and extended with a sandbag to hold the feet in place (Figs. 10.3 and 10.4).

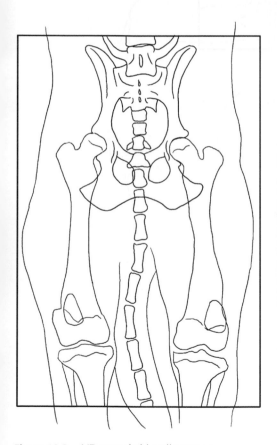

Figure 10.3.   VD extended leg illustration.

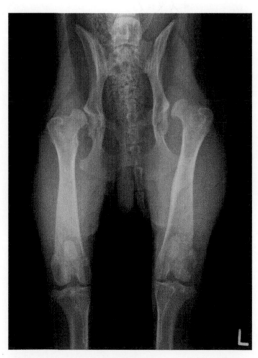

Figure 10.4.   VD extended leg.

CHAPTER 10

View: Ventrodorsal Frog-Leg

Place the patient in dorsal recumbent position with the head in a head cradle positioning sponge with the Head End against the shoulders. Make sure the sternum and spine are superimposed as the hind legs are left in the normal flexed position. The femur should be at an approximately 45-degree angle to the spine. Sandbags or masking tape over the tarsal joints will hold the legs in position (Figs. 10.5 through 10.7).

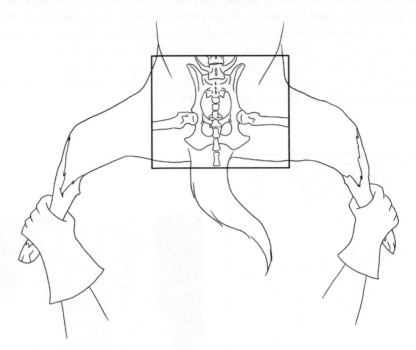

Figure 10.5.   VD frog-leg illustration.

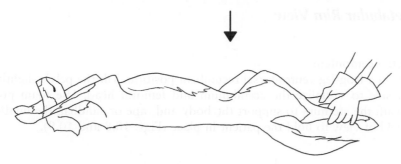

Figure 10.6.   VD frog-leg illustration side view.

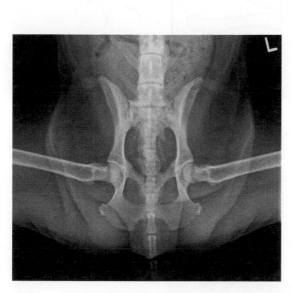

Figure 10.7.   VD frog-leg view.

View: *Acetabular Rim View*

Center Point: Acetabulum.

Place patient in a frog-leg ventrodorsal recumbent position. Tilt the pelvis slightly toward the affected side to visualize the acetabulum and femoral head. Use foam positioning wedges beneath the sternum to support the body and tape or sandbag the unaffected leg out of the field of view to hold the patient in place (Figs. 10.8 and 10.9).

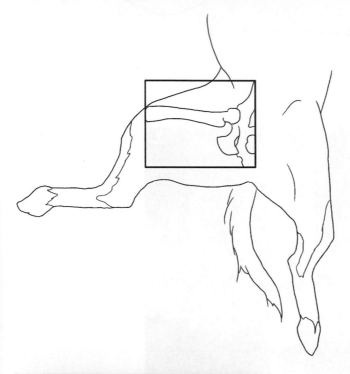

Figure 10.8. Acetabular rim illustration.

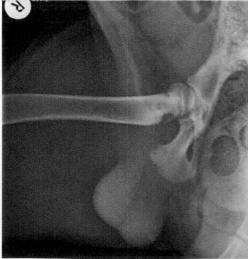

Figure 10.9. Acetabular rim view.

OFA Imaging

Information regarding OFA imaging and submission instructions was retrieved from the Orthopedic Foundation for Animals' website (http://www.offa.org/hd_procedures.html). Radiographs submitted to the OFA should follow the American Veterinary Medical Association recommendations for positioning. This view is accepted worldwide for detection and assessment of hip joint irregularities and secondary arthritic hip joint changes. To obtain this view, the animal must be placed on its back in a dorsal recumbent position with the rear limbs extended and parallel to each other. The stifles are rotated internally and the pelvis is symmetric. Chemical restraint (anesthesia) to the point of relaxation is recommended but not required. With chemical restraint, optimum patient positioning is easier with minimal repeat radiographs and a truer representation of the hip status is obtained. For elbows, the animal is placed on its side and the respective elbow is placed in an extreme flexed position (Figs. 10.10 and 10.11).

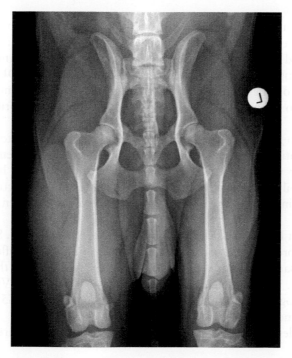

Figure 10.10.   OFA pelvis extended leg.

CHAPTER 10

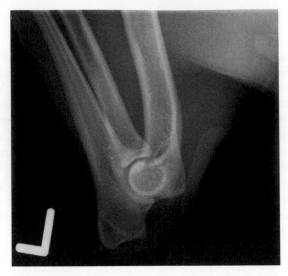

Figure 10.11.   OFA hyperflexed elbow.

The radiograph film must be permanently identified with the animal's registration number or name, date the radiograph was taken, and the veterinarian's name or hospital name. If this required information is illegible or missing, the OFA cannot accept the film for registration purposes. The owner should complete and sign the OFA application. It is important to record on the OFA application the animal's tattoo or microchip number in order for the OFA to submit results to the AKC. Sire and dam information should also be present.

Radiography of pregnant or estrus females should be avoided due to possible increased joint laxity (subluxation) from hormonal variations. OFA recommends radiographs be taken 1 month after weaning pups and 1 month before or after a heat cycle. Physical inactivity because of illness, weather, or the owner's management practices may also result in some degree of joint laxity. The OFA recommends evaluation when the dog is in good physical condition.

For large and giant breed dogs, 14″ × 17″ film size is recommended. Small film sizes can be used for smaller breeds if the area between the sacrum and the stifles can be included.

If a copy is necessary ask your veterinarian to insert two films in the cassette prior to making the exposure. This will require about a 15% increase in the kVp to make an exact duplicate of the radiograph sent to OFA. Films may be returned if a $5.00 fee and request for return are both included at time of submission.

Good contrast is desirable (high mAs, low kVp). Grid techniques are recommended for all large dogs.

Radiation Safety

Proper collimation and protection of attendants is the responsibility of the veterinarian. Gonadal shielding is recommended for male dogs.

Mailing Recommendations

The radiograph, application, and fees should be enclosed in a mailing envelope. These may be paper clipped together. Use the mail service of your choice. Obtain large envelopes from an office supply store, veterinary hospital, or other radiology department. The envelope should be sealed with tape. Light cardboard may be included to stiffen the package but is not required. Avoid using boxes, tubes, padded envelopes, stapling check and application, bending/folding radiographs, or taping application or check to envelope.

OFA's Handling Procedures

When a radiograph arrives at the OFA, the information on the radiograph is checked against information on the application. The age of the dog is calculated, and the submitted fee is recorded. The board-certified veterinary radiologist on staff at the OFA screens the radiograph for diagnostic quality. If it is not suitable for diagnostic quality (poor positioning, too light, too dark, or image blurring from motion), it is returned to the referring veterinarian with a written request that it be repeated. An application number is assigned.

PennHIP Information

PennHIP is the most accurate hip screening method available and can be safely performed on dogs as young as 16 weeks of age. Veterinarians must attend a training seminar to learn how to position the PennHIP projections. They must personally position for these studies, though one of their staff can also be trained to perform the studies if the staff member accompanies the veterinarian to the training seminar to also be trained. When they return to their respective practices, the PennHIP veterinarians (and veterinary technicians, if applicable) will each have to submit three sets of PennHIP radiographs to the University of Pennsylvania before they can officially become certified to perform this study at their practice. An early estimate of a dog's hip integrity is invaluable, whether the dog's intended purpose is for breeding, for working, or as a family pet. For breeders, information compiled in PennHIP's international database permits informed selection of breeding stock based on hip tightness relative to other members of the same breed. Breeders can reduce the incidence and severity of canine hip dysplasia (CHD) in future generations of dogs by applying selection pressure toward tighter hips. Among current hip screening methods, PennHIP has the highest heritability value to bring about these genetic changes. Service and working dog organizations use PennHIP as the principal method for hip screening. The investment in training service/working dogs is enormous. The ability to prescreen the dog's genetic predisposition to CHD is an invaluable tool when evaluating a future service/working dog's hip integrity. For companion dog owners, if the dog is identified to be at risk for CHD, the PennHIP veterinarian can recommend, at an early age, appropriate strategies (diet, medication, and/or activities) to delay or diminish the ultimate course of the disease.

CHAPTER 10

The PennHIP veterinarian will submit the three PennHIP radiographs to the University of Pennsylvania for specialized evaluation (for examples, see Figs. 10.12 through 10.14). A confidential report will be sent to the owner and the PennHIP veterinarian: The distraction index (DI) is a measure of hip laxity—the inherent distance the ball can be displaced (distracted) from the hip socket—and is expressed as a number between 0 and 1. A DI near zero indicates little joint laxity (very tight hips). A DI closer to 1.0 indicates a high degree of laxity (very loose hips). Dogs with tighter hips are less likely to develop hip dysplasia than dogs with looser hips. A threshold level of 0.30 has been identified, below which hip dysplasia is very unlikely to occur. The PennHIP report also includes an evaluation of the hip-extended radiograph for evidence of arthritis, confirming a diagnosis of hip dysplasia. Based on the DI, the dog is ranked within its breed. For the dog breeder this ranking helps in the selection of breeding candidates—dogs in the tighter half of the population are recommended for breeding. By selecting breeding

CHAPTER 10

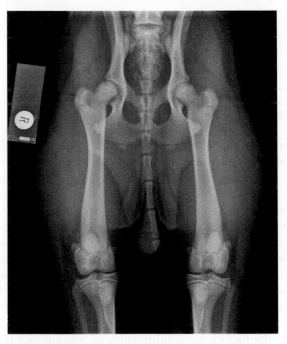

Figure 10.12.   PennHIP VD extended leg pelvis.

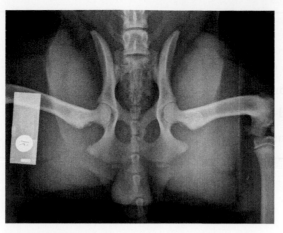

Figure 10.13. PennHIP compression view.

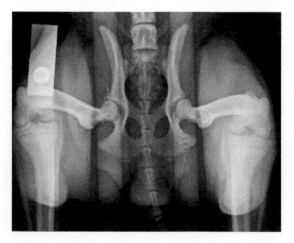

Figure 10.14. PennHIP distraction view.

dogs with tight hips (lower DI), meaningful progress toward better hips can be made within a few generations. For more detailed information, visit the PennHIP website at www.pennhip.org.

PennHIP
The University of Pennsylvania
School of Veterinary Medicine
3800 Spruce Street
Philadelphia, Pennsylvania 19104

Femur

The routine views of the femur are CrCd and lateral views.

Sedation: Recommended.

Center Point: Mid-shaft of the femur.

Measurement Point: Mid-shaft of the femur.

View: Lateral View

Place the patient in a lateral recumbent position, affected side down. Flex and move the unaffected leg out of the field of view. Use tape and/or a sandbag to secure the unaffected leg. Placing gauze or a thin foam pad beneath the proximal tibia will prevent rotation of the femur. Include the hip and stifle joint in the field of view (Figs. 10.15 and 10.16).

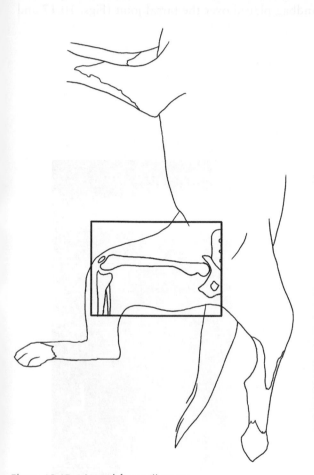

Figure 10.15.   Lateral femur illustration.

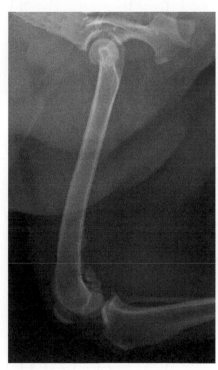

Figure 10.16.   Lateral femur.

View: Craniocaudal View

Place the patient in dorsal recumbent position with the patient's head in a head cradle positioning sponge with the Head End immobilization device or two sandbags against the shoulders. Extend the affected leg caudally and abduct slightly to remove superimposition of the tuber ischium. The femur should be as parallel as possible to the tabletop with the patella positioned between the femoral condyles. The field of view should include both the hip and stifle joints. The unaffected leg should be flexed and rotated laterally out of the field of view and secured with a sandbag placed over the tarsal joint (Figs. 10.17 and 10.18).

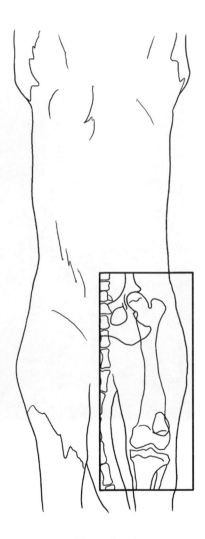

Figure 10.17.   CrCd femur illustration.

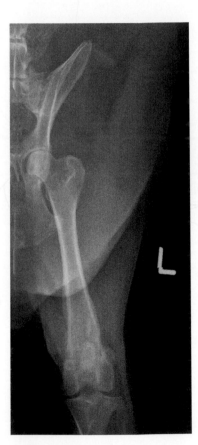

Figure 10.18.   CrCd femur.

Stifle

The routine views for the stifle joint are caudocranial and lateral views. For the lateral view of the stifle, some veterinarians prefer a 90-degree flexed lateral over the more natural slightly flexed lateral, particularly in specialty practices. Supplemental view: Skyline (sunrise or tangential) view of the patella. This tangential view evaluates the depth of the trochlear groove and demonstrates the femoropatellar joint space.

Sedation: Recommended.

Center Point: Stifle joint.

Measurement Point: Distal femur.

View: Lateral View

The patient is placed in a lateral recumbent position with the unaffected leg moved laterally and secured outside the field of view with tape or sandbag. Alternate positioning technique has the unaffected leg pulled cranially, ventral to the abdomen, and secured with sandbag, tape, or Head End immobilization device. Smaller dogs, cats, or dogs with short legs are more easily positioned for the lateral view if the unaffected leg is flexed, moved laterally, and secured outside the field of view. The affected stifle joint is flexed either 90 degrees or a more natural slightly flexed angle, usually 60 degrees, clinician preference. Place gauze or small thin positioning foam beneath the calcaneous to ensure the tibia is parallel to the tabletop or cassette and the femoral condyles are superimposed (Figs. 10.19 through 10.21).

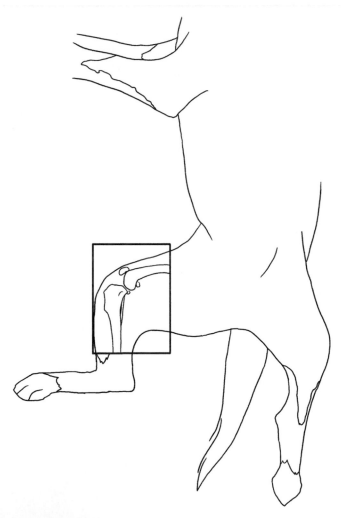

Figure 10.19.   Lateral view illustration.

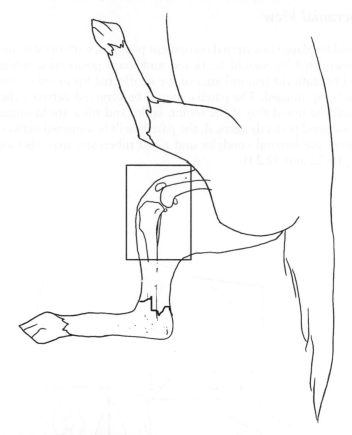

Figure 10.20.   Lateral view alternate illustration.

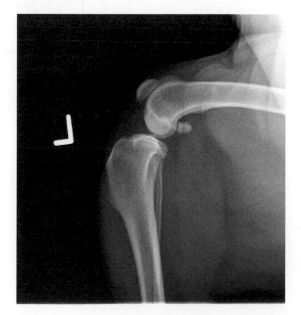

Figure 10.21.   Lateral view.

View: Caudocranial View

The patient should be placed in a sternal recumbent position, with the affected leg extended caudally. The unaffected leg should be flexed and foam positioning wedge or sandbag should be placed beneath the femoral area of the unaffected leg to aid in controlling rotation of the stifle being imaged. The patella should be centered between the two femoral condyles. It should be noted that if the femur, stifle, and tibia are in alignment and the calcaneous is positioned perfectly vertical, the patella will be centered between the femoral condyles. Palpating the femoral condyles and tibial tuberosity may also aid in checking symmetry (Figs. 10.22 and 10.23).

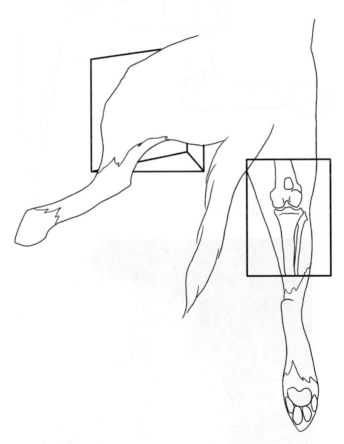

Figure 10.22.   CdCr view illustration.

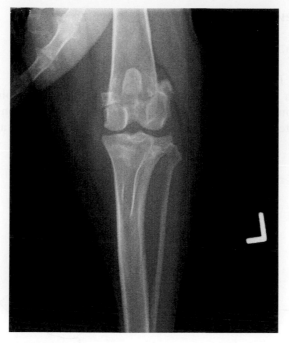

Figure 10.23.   CdCr view.

View: Skyline View

Center Point: Patella.

Measurement Point: Patella.

Place the patient in a sternal recumbent position with the affected joint fully flexed with the distal extremity pulled caudally. X-ray beam should be centered on the patella and the field of view collimated to include the femoral condyles (Figs. 10.24 and 10.25).

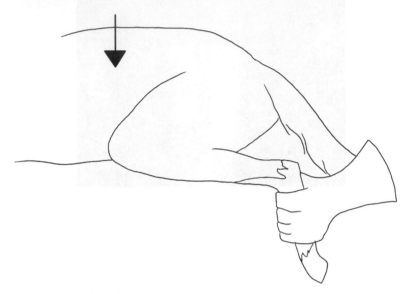

Figure 10.24.   Sunrise view of patella illustration.

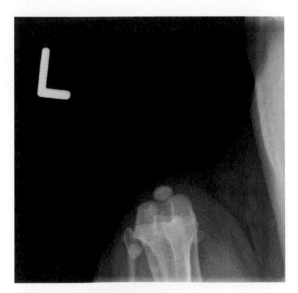

Figure 10.25.   Sunrise view of patella.

Tibial Plateau Leveling Osteotomy (TPLO)

The TPLO is a surgical technique developed to treat cranial cruciate ligament tears in dogs. The routine views are CdCr and lateral views of the tibia. The lateral view requires both the stifle and tarsal joints to be flexed 90 degrees.

Sedation: Recommended.

Center Point: Middle of tibia.

Measurement Point: Stifle.

CHAPTER 10

View: Lateral View

The patient is placed in a lateral recumbent position with the unaffected leg moved laterally and secured outside the field of view with tape or sandbag. Alternate positioning technique has the unaffected leg pulled cranially, ventral to the abdomen, and secured with sandbag, tape, or Head End immobilization device. The stifle and tarsal joints are flexed 90 degrees. Place gauze or small thin positioning foam beneath the calcaneous to ensure the tibia is parallel to the tabletop or cassette and the femoral condyles are superimposed. Both the stifle and tarsal joints should be in the field of view (Figs. 10.26 through 10.28).

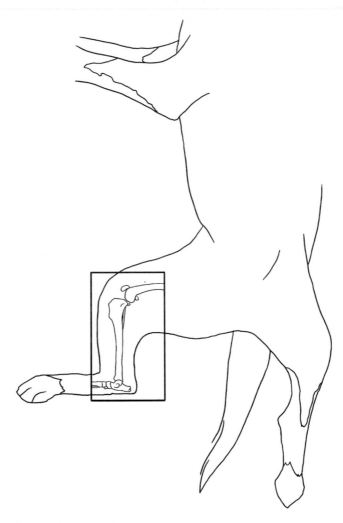

Figure 10.26.   Lateral TPLO view illustration.

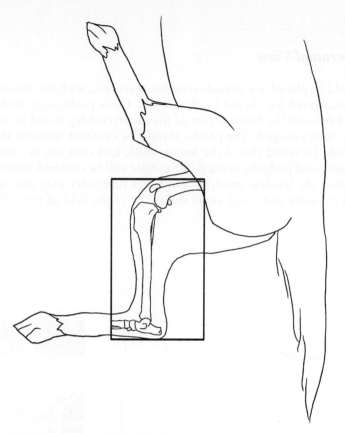

Figure 10.27. Lateral TPLO view alternate illustration.

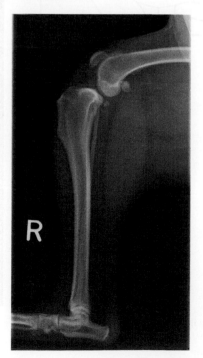

R

Figure 10.28. Lateral TPLO view.

View: Caudocranial View

The patient should be placed in a sternal recumbent position, with the affected leg extended caudally. The unaffected leg should be flexed and foam positioning wedge or sandbag should be placed beneath the femoral area of the unaffected leg to aid in controlling rotation of the stifle being imaged. The patella should be centered between the two femoral condyles. It should be noted that if the femur, stifle, and tibia are in alignment and the calcaneous is positioned perfectly vertical, the patella will be centered between the femoral condyles. Palpating the femoral condyles and tibial tuberosity may also aid in checking symmetry. Both the stifle and tarsal joints should be in the field of view (Figs. 10.29 and 10.30).

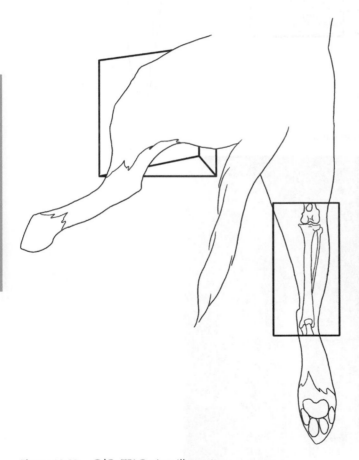

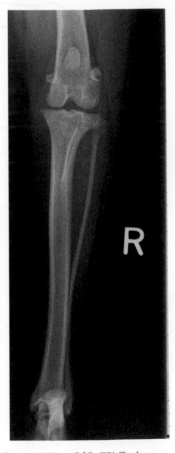

Figure 10.29.   CdCr TPLO view illustration.   Figure 10.30.   CdCr TPLO view.

Tibial Tuberosity Advancement (TTA)

The TTA is a surgical technique developed to correct a rupture of the cranial cruciate ligament (CCL), also referred to as the anterior cruciate ligament (ACL). The routine views taken are lateral and CdCr views of the stifle.

Center Point: Stifle joint.

Measurement Point: Distal femur.

View: *Lateral View*

The patient is placed in a lateral recumbent position with the unaffected leg moved laterally and secured outside the field of view with tape or sandbag. Center the beam on the stifle joint space. The tibia should be positioned in true lateral, as parallel and close to the tabletop as possible to decrease magnification (< 5%). Place gauze or thin positioning foam beneath the calcaneous to help ensure the femoral condyles are superimposed. The femorotibial angle should be 135 degrees, to mimic the normal canine standing stance. The collimated field of view should include the mid diaphyses of the femur and tibia. For post-op images, the field of view should include the total implant (Figs. 10.31 and 10.32).

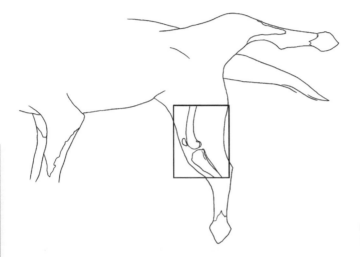

Figure 10.31.   Lateral TTA view illustration.

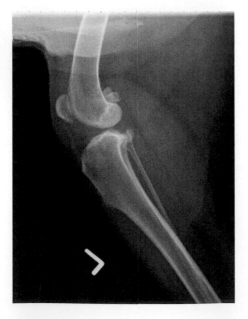

Figure 10.32.   Lateral TTA view.

View: Caudocranial View

The patient is placed in a sternal recumbent position, with the affected leg extended caudally. The unaffected leg should be flexed and foam positioning wedge or sandbag should be placed beneath the femoral area of the unaffected leg to aid in controlling rotation of the stifle being imaged. The patella should be centered between the two femoral condyles. It should be noted that if the femur, stifle, and tibia are in alignment and the calcaneous is positioned perfectly vertical, the patella will be centered between the femoral condyles. Palpating the femoral condyles and tibial tuberosity may also aid in checking symmetry. The collimated field of view includes the mid-diaphyses of the femur and tibia. For postoperative images, the field of view should include the entire implant (Figs. 10.33 and 10.34).

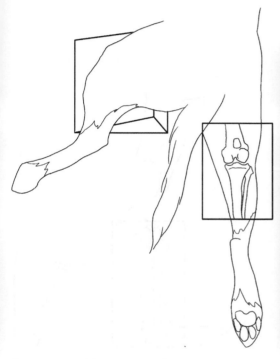

Figure 10.33.   CdCr TTA view illustration.

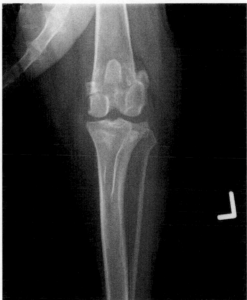

Figure 10.34.   CdCr TTA view.

Tibia and Fibula

The routine views for tibia and fibula are CdCr and lateral views.

Sedation: Recommended.

Center Point: Middle of tibia.

Measurement Point: Stifle.

View: Lateral View

The patient is placed in a lateral recumbent position with the unaffected leg moved laterally and secured outside the field of view with tape or sandbag. Alternate positioning technique has the unaffected leg pulled cranially, ventral to the abdomen, and secured with sandbag, tape, or Head End immobilization device. The stifle and tarsal joints are flexed 90 degrees. Place gauze or small thin positioning foam beneath the calcaneous to ensure the tibia is parallel to the tabletop or cassette and the femoral condyles are superimposed. Both the stifle and tarsal joints should be in the field of view (Figs. 10.35a and b and 10.36).

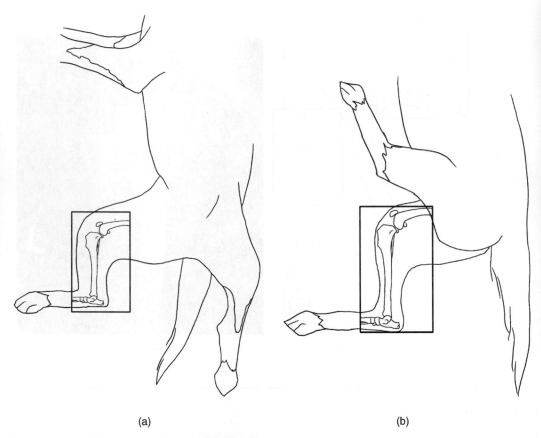

(a)   (b)

Figure 10.35a and b.   Lateral tibia view illustrations.

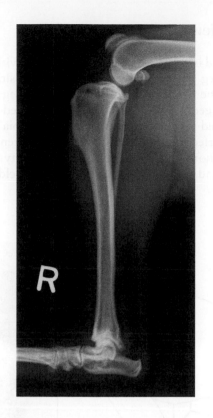

Figure 10.36. Lateral tibia.

View: Caudocranial View

The patient should be placed in a sternal recumbent position, with the affected leg extended caudally. The unaffected leg should be flexed and foam positioning wedge or sandbag should be placed beneath the femoral area of the unaffected leg to aid in controlling rotation of the stifle being imaged. The patella should be centered between the two femoral condyles. It should be noted that if the femur, stifle, and tibia are in alignment and the calcaneous is positioned perfectly vertical, the patella will be centered between the femoral condyles. Palpating the femoral condyles and tibial tuberosity may also aid in checking symmetry. Both the stifle and tarsal joints should be in the field of view (Figs. 10.37 and 10.38).

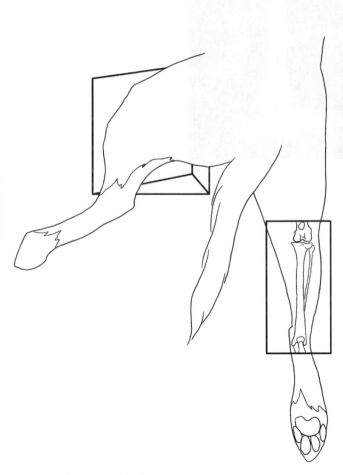

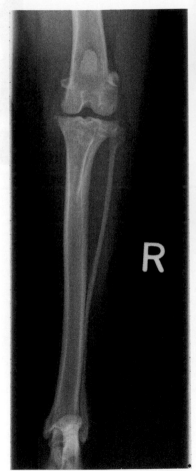

Figure 10.37.   CdCr tibia illustration.

Figure 10.38.   CdCr tibia.

Tarsus

Routine views of the tarsus are dorsoplantar and lateral views. Supplemental views are flexion, extension, oblique, and stress views.

Sedation: Recommended.

Center Point: Tarsal joint.

Measurement Point: Tarsal joint.

View: Lateral View

The patient is placed in a lateral recumbent position with the unaffected leg moved laterally and secured outside the field of view with tape or sandbag. Alternate positioning technique has the unaffected leg pulled cranially, ventral to the abdomen, and secured with sandbag, tape, or Head End immobilization device. The tarsal joint can be flexed 90 degrees or left in a natural flexed position, clinician's preference. Place gauze or small thin positioning foam beneath the calcaneous to ensure the tibia is parallel to the tabletop. Collimate so the distal tibia and fibula and metatarsal bones are in the field of view (Figs. 10.39 and 10.40).

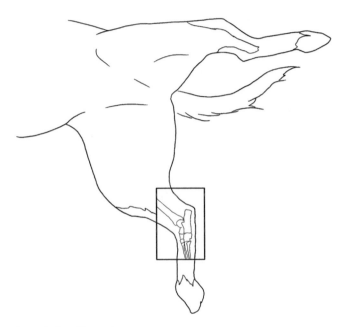

Figure 10.39.   Lateral tarsal view illustration.

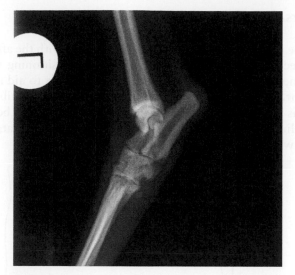

Figure 10.40.   Lateral tarsal view.

View: Plantardorsal or Dorsoplantar Views

The patient should be placed in a sternal recumbent position, with the affected leg extended caudally. The unaffected leg should be flexed and foam positioning wedge or sandbag should be placed beneath the femoral area of the unaffected leg to aid in controlling rotation of the tarsal joint. It should be noted that if the femur, stifle, and tibia are in alignment and the calcaneous is positioned perfectly vertical, the tarsus should be in a true plantardorsal position. Collimate so the distal tibia and fibula and the metatarsal bones should be in the field of view (Figs. 10.41 and 10.42).

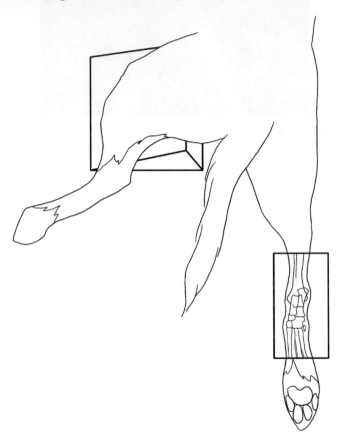

Figure 10.41.   Plantardorsal tarsal view illustration.

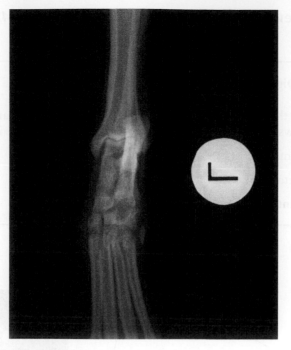

Figure 10.42. Plantardorsal tarsus.

Supplemental Views: Oblique and Stress Views (Figs. 10.43 and 10.44)

Metatarsus and Digits

Routine views of the metatarsus and phalanges are dorsoplantar and lateral views. Supplemental views are oblique views and lateral views to offset the individual digits.

Sedation: Recommended.

Center Point: Metatarsal bones.

Measurement Point: Metatarsal bones.

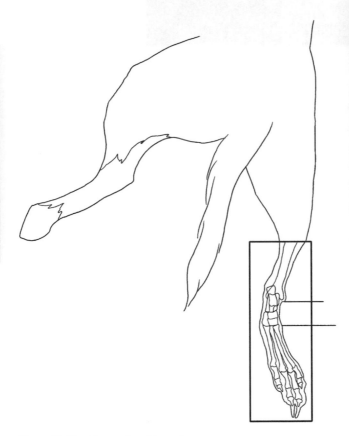

Figure 10.43.　Stress view illustration.

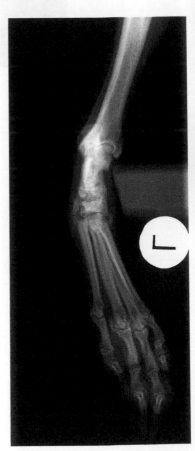

Figure 10.44.　Tarsal stress view.

View: Lateral View

The patient is placed in a lateral recumbent position with the unaffected leg moved laterally and secured outside the field of view with tape or sandbag. Alternate positioning technique has the unaffected leg pulled cranially, ventral to the abdomen, and secured with sandbag, tape, or Head End immobilization device. The metatarsal bones are left in a natural flexed position. Place gauze or small thin positioning foam beneath the calcaneous to ensure the foot is parallel to the tabletop. Collimate so the distal tibia and fibula and the tips of the digits are in the field of view (Figs. 10.45 and 10.46).

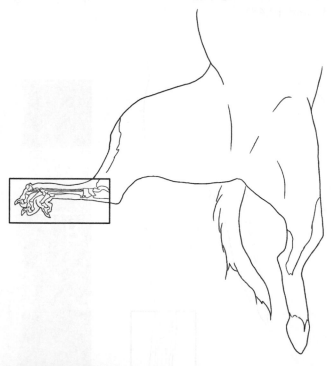

Figure 10.45. Lateral metatarsal view illustration.

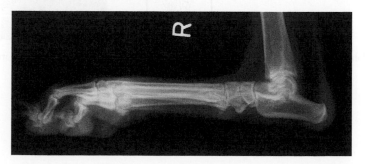

Figure 10.46. Lateral metatarsus with digits.

CHAPTER 10

View: *Plantardorsal or Dorsoplantar Views*

The patient should be placed in a sternal recumbent position, with the affected leg extended caudally. The unaffected leg should be flexed and foam positioning wedge or sandbag should be placed beneath the femoral area of the unaffected leg to aid in controlling rotation of the tarsal joint. It should be noted that if the femur, stifle, and tibia are in alignment and the calcaneous is positioned perfectly vertical, the tarsus and metatarsus should be in a true plantardorsal position. Collimate so the field of view should include the distal tibia and fibula and the tips of the digits. An alternate position is the dorsoplantar (DPl) view, where the affected leg is extended cranially, next to the body. Center over the metatarsal bones and collimate so the distal tibia and fibula and the tips of the digits are in the field of view (Figs. 10.47 and 10.48).

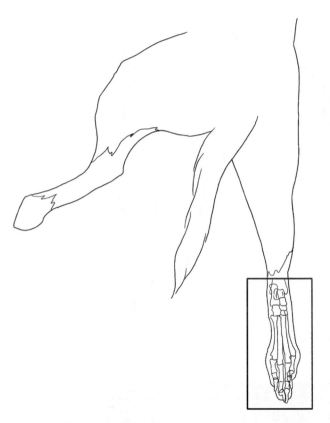

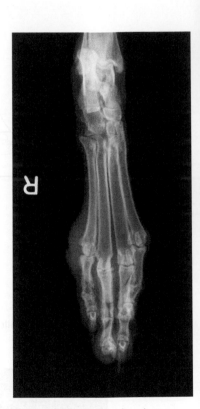

Figure 10.47.　Plantardorsal illustration.

Figure 10.48.　Plantardorsal view.

Supplemental Views: Oblique Views (Figs. 10.49 and 10.50)

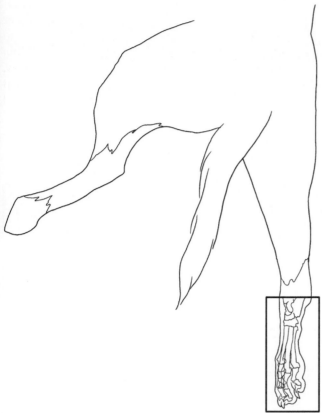

Figure 10.49.   Metatarsal oblique illustration.

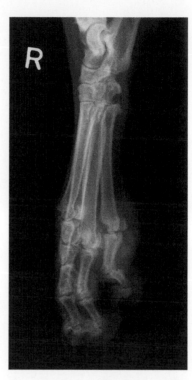

Figure 10.50.   Metatarsal oblique.

Small Animal Positioning—Spine

Spinal imaging requires careful positioning. The divergence of the x-ray beam and the importance of imaging the intervertebral disc spaces require the spine to be as parallel to the tabletop as possible. This can be achieved by using radiolucent foam positioning wedges and imaging the spine in short segments. Centering and collimating to the spinal area of interest will help minimize the geometric distortion and the scattered radiation produced. A grid is recommended for imaging the spinal column. Heavy sedation or general anesthesia is preferred for imaging studies of the spine. Supplemental views such as flexion, extension, and oblique views may be requested by the veterinarian. Flexion and extension views should be done under direct supervision of the clinician, particularly when a fracture, luxation, or other instability is suspected. Contrast studies of the spine performed under general anesthesia include myelography and epidurography (Figs. 11.1 and 11.2).

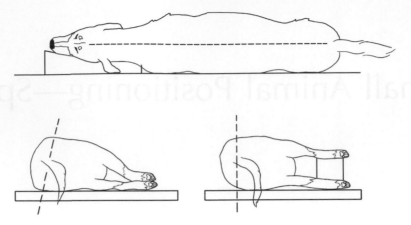

Figure 11.1.   Spinal lateral positioning diagram.

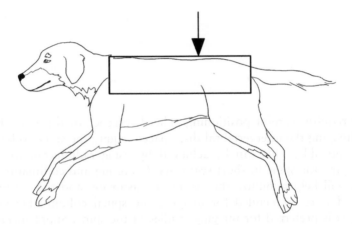

Figure 11.2.   Spinal lateral positioning diagram 2.

Cervical Spine

The cervical spine consists of seven cervical vertebrae. C1 and C2 are referred to as the atlas and the axis, respectively. The odontoid process is part of C2. C6 has large transverse processes. The routine imaging views are ventrodorsal (VD) and lateral views. Supplemental views include flexion, extension, open mouth view of the odontoid process, and oblique views. When looking for cervical instability, the veterinarian should determine the degree of flexion to be used.

Sedation: Recommended; general anesthesia preferred to attain best-quality images of the spine.

Center Point: Mid-cervical.

Measurement Point: Caudal cervical over shoulder joints.

View: Lateral View

Place the patient in a lateral recumbent position with the head extended. The position of the head affects the obliquity of the spine. Place a wedge beneath the nose, and if the mid-cervical area appears to be sagging, place a flat piece of positioning foam to keep the spine parallel to the tabletop. The forelimbs should be extended caudally toward the abdomen (Figs. 11.3 and 11.4).

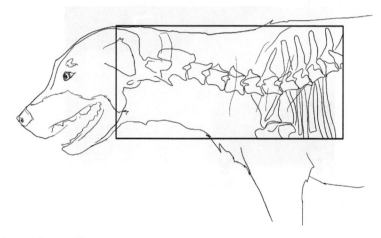

Figure 11.3.   Lateral C spine illustration.

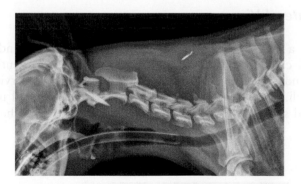

Figure 11.4.   Lateral C spine.

View: Extension Lateral View

Place the patient in a lateral recumbent position with the head extended. The forelimbs should be extended caudally toward the abdomen. The head is gently moved dorsally and a positioning wedge placed beneath the mandible to reduce obliquity of the skull and reinforced by a sandbag positioned against the wedge to hold both in place. The extension view should always be done first, evaluated by the veterinarian before positioning for the flexion view (Fig. 11.5).

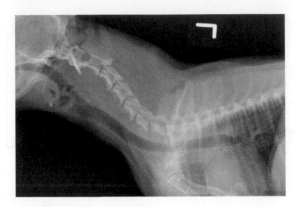

Figure 11.5.   Lateral C spine extension.

View: Flexion Lateral View

Place the patient in a lateral recumbent position with the head extended. The forelimbs should be extended caudally toward the abdomen. The head is gently pulled caudally toward the thorax and positioning foam placed beneath the cranial cervical spine to reduce obliquity of the skull. The head can be pulled caudally and secured using roll gauze or manually pulled and secured with a Head End or sandbag to hold the head and neck in place (Fig. 11.6).

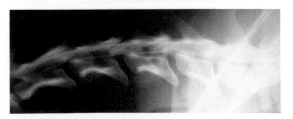

Figure 11.6.   Lateral C spine flexion.

View: Ventrodorsal View

Place the patient in a dorsal recumbent position with the patient's nose directed slightly upward to minimize curving the cervical spine. The forelegs are pulled caudally and secured with tape. The patient should be in a true VD position with the sternum and spine superimposed and the cervical spine parallel to the tabletop. The field of view should include the base of the skull and the second thoracic vertebra (Figs. 11.7 and 11.8).

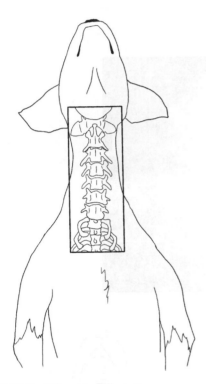

Figure 11.7. VD cervical illustration.

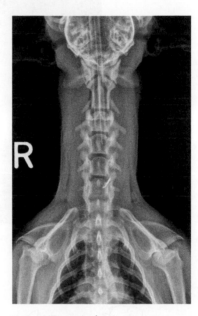

Figure 11.8. VD cervical spine.

View: Open Mouth Ventrodorsal View of the Odontoid

Place the patient in a dorsal recumbent position with the patient's nose directed upward and the mouth opened by using either gauze or masking tape to pull the maxillary arcade slightly cranial and the mandible caudally. The commissure of the lips should be positioned over C2. The forelegs are pulled caudally and secured with tape. The patient should be in a true VD position with the sternum and spine superimposed and the cervical spine parallel to the tabletop. The endotracheal tube should be removed or tied to the mandible. Center over C2 (Figs. 11.9a through 11.9c).

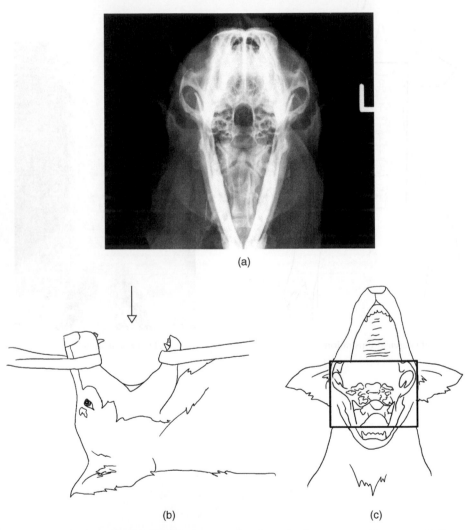

(a)

(b)   (c)

Figure 11.9.   (a) Open mouth odontoid. (b) Open mouth odontoid side projection illustration. (c) Open mouth odontoid frontal projection illustration.

CHAPTER 11

Thoracic Spine and Thoraco-Lumbar Spine

The thoracic spine consists of 13 vertebrae, articulating with ribs. The routine views for thoracic spine are VD and lateral views. If imaging a cat or small-to-medium dog, the lumbar spine is included in the field of view. There are 7 lumbar vertebrae.

Sedation: Recommended.

Center Point: Thoracic Spine: Mid-thoracic spine.

Center Point: TL Spine: TL junction.

Measurement Point: Highest point of the ribs.

View: *Lateral View*

Place the patient in a lateral recumbent position with the fore and hind legs moderately extended cranially and caudally, respectively. Place a foam positioning wedge beneath the sternum to ensure the spine is positioned in a true lateral projection. The spine and sternum should be parallel to each other. If imaging the lumbar spine, another foam positioning wedge may be needed beneath the abdomen to reduce obliquity of the lumbar vertebrae. For thoracic spine, collimate the field of view to include C7 through L1. For TL spine, collimate the field to include C7 to S1 (Figs. 11.10 through 11.13).

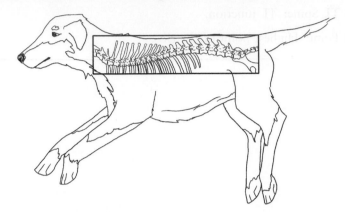

Figure 11.10.   Lateral TL spine illustration.

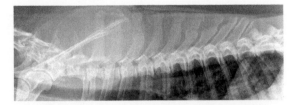

Figure 11.11.   Lateral thoracic spine large dog.

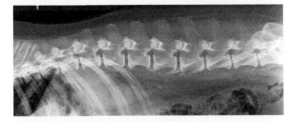

Figure 11.12.   Lateral caudal TL spine large dog.

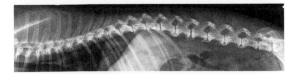

Figure 11.13.   Lateral TL spine.

View: Ventrodorsal View

Place the patient in a dorsal recumbent position with the forelegs extended cranially and secured with tape and the hind legs extended slightly caudally and positioned in a frog position to ensure the spine is parallel to the tabletop. Sandbags or a Head End patient immobilization device may be used to support the patient's shoulders, preventing the body from tilting side to side. Placing a sandbag on either side of the patient at the pelvis will help keep the patient in a true VD position and also support the frogged hind legs. The sternum should be superimposed over the thoracic spine. For thoracic spine, collimate the field of view to include C7 through L1. For TL spine, collimate the field to include C7 to S1 (Figs. 11.14 through 11.17).

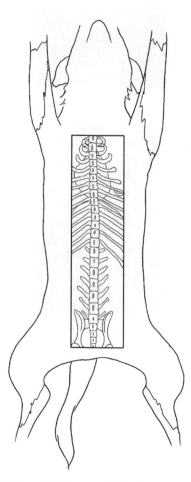

Figure 11.14.   VD TL spine illustration.

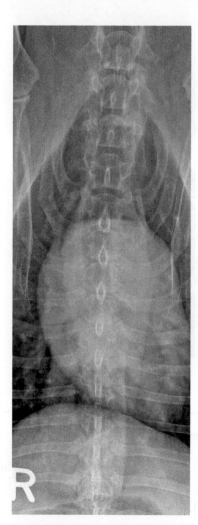

Figure 11.15.   VD thoracic spine large dog.

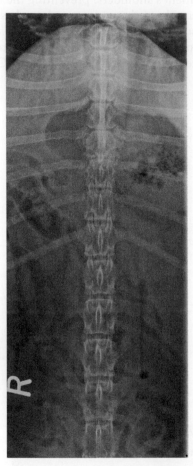

Figure 11.16.   VD TL caudal large dog.

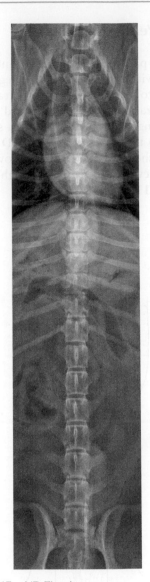

Figure 11.17.   VD TL spine.

Lumbar Spine

The lumbar spine consists of seven lumbar vertebrae. The routine views for imaging the lumbar spine area are VD and lateral views.

Sedation: Recommended.

Center Point: Mid-lumbar region.

Measurement Point: Cranial lumbar region.

View: Lateral View

Place the patient in a lateral recumbent position with the fore and hind legs moderately extended cranially and caudally, respectively. Place a foam positioning wedge beneath the sternum to ensure the spine is positioned in a true lateral projection. The spine and sternum should be parallel to each other. Another foam positioning wedge may be needed beneath the abdomen to reduce obliquity of the lumbar vertebrae. Collimate to include T13 to S1 in the field of view (Figs. 11.18 and 11.19).

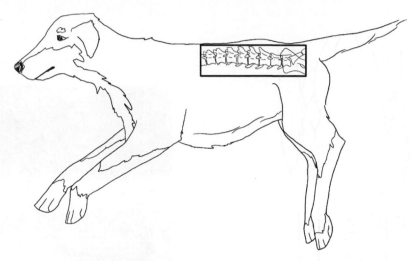

Figure 11.18.   Lateral L spine illustration.

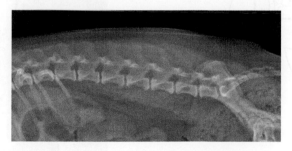

Figure 11.19.   Lateral lumbar spine.

View: Ventrodorsal View

Place the patient in a dorsal recumbent position with the forelegs extended cranially and secured with tape and the hind legs extended slightly caudally and positioned in a flexed frog position to ensure the spine is parallel to the tabletop. Sandbags or a Head End patient immobilization device may be used to support the patient's shoulders, preventing the body from tilting side to side. Placing a sandbag on either side of the patient at the pelvis will help keep the patient in a true VD position and also support the frogged hind limbs. The sternum should be superimposed over the thoracic spine (Figs. 11.20 and 11.21).

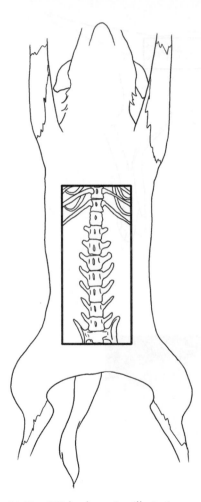

Figure 11.20.   VD lumbar spine illustration.

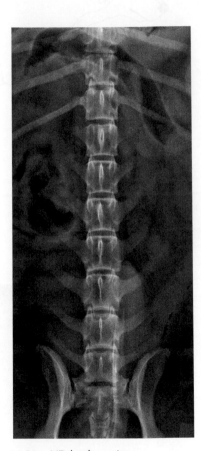

Figure 11.21.   VD lumbar spine.

LS Spine

The routine views for imaging the lumbosacral spine are ventrodorsal, neutral, flexed, and extended lateral views of the lumbosacral junction. The views are typically used to demonstrate lumbar stenosis or are taken in conjunction with myelography.

Sedation: Recommended.

Center Point: Lumbosacral junction.

Measurement Point: Lumbosacral junction.

View: Neutral Lateral

Place the patient in a lateral recumbent position with the fore and hind legs moderately extended cranially and caudally, respectively. Place a foam positioning wedge beneath the sternum to ensure the spine is positioned in a true lateral projection. The spine and sternum should be parallel to each other. Another foam positioning wedge may be needed beneath the abdomen to reduce obliquity of the lumbar vertebrae. Collimate to include L4 to S3 in the field of view (Figs. 11.22 and 11.23).

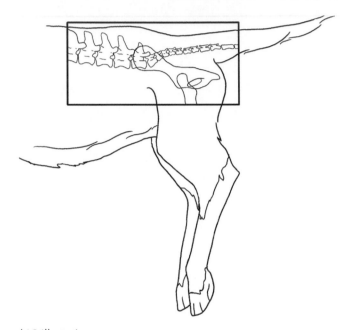

Figure 11.22.   Lateral LS illustration.

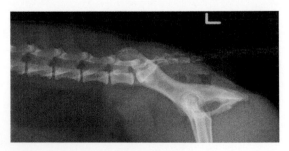

Figure 11.23.   Lateral LS spine.

View: Extended Lateral

Place the patient in a lateral recumbent position with the fore and hind legs moderately extended cranially. Place a foam positioning wedge beneath the sternum to ensure the spine is positioned in a true lateral projection. The spine and sternum should be parallel to each other. Another foam positioning wedge may be needed beneath the abdomen to reduce obliquity of the lumbar vertebrae. Gently move the hind legs caudodorsally, minimizing movement of the upper body. Collimate to include L4 to S3 in the field of view (Figs. 11.24 and 11.25).

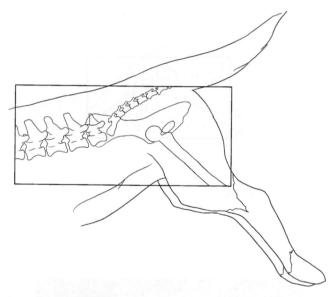

Figure 11.24. Lateral LS extension illustration.

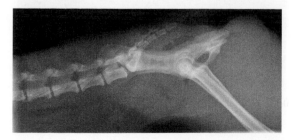

Figure 11.25. Lateral LS extension.

View: Flexed Lateral

Place the patient in a lateral recumbent position with the fore and hind legs moderately extended cranially and caudally, respectively. Place a foam positioning wedge beneath the sternum to ensure the spine is positioned in a true lateral projection. The spine and sternum should be parallel to each other. Gently pull the hind legs cranially, flexing the LS spine while minimizing movement of the upper body. Collimate to include L4 to S3 in the field of view (Figs. 11.26 and 11.27).

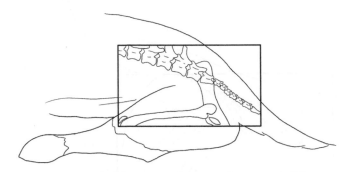

Figure 11.26.   Lateral LS flexion illustration.

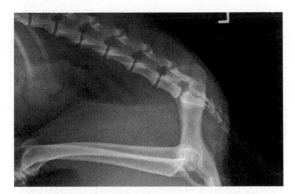

Figure 11.27.   Lateral LS flexion.

View: Ventrodorsal View

Place the patient in a dorsal recumbent position with the forelegs extended cranially and secured with tape and the hind legs extended slightly caudally and positioned in a relaxed position. Sandbags or a Head End patient immobilization device may be used to support the patient's shoulders, preventing the body from tilting side to side. The sternum should be superimposed over the thoracic spine. Collimate the field of view to include L4 through S3 (Figs. 11.28 and 11.29).

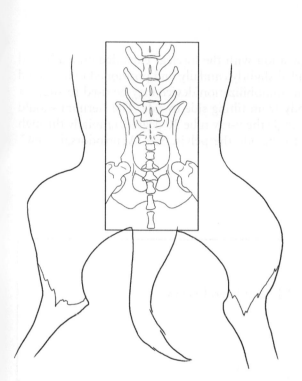

Figure 11.28.   VD LS spine illustration.

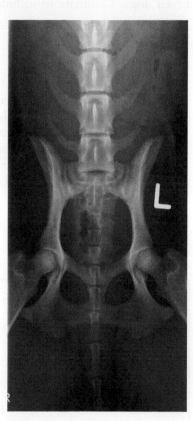

Figure 11.29.   VD LS spine.

CHAPTER 11

Sacrum

The routine views for visualizing the sacrum are lateral and a 30-degree angle toward the head through the sacrum.

Sedation: Recommended.

Center Point: Sacrum.

Measurement Point: Sacrum.

View: Lateral View

Place the patient in a lateral recumbent position with the fore and hind legs moderately extended cranially and caudally, respectively. Place a foam positioning wedge beneath the sternum to ensure the spine is positioned in a true lateral projection. The spine and sternum should be parallel to each other. Another foam positioning wedge may be needed beneath the abdomen to reduce obliquity of the lumbar vertebrae. The tuber ischii should be superimposed. Sometimes a positioning wedge is needed between the hind legs for larger breed dogs. Collimate to include the pelvis in the field of view. See "LS Spine," lateral views.

View: Ventrodorsal View

Place the patient in a dorsal recumbent position with the forelegs extended cranially and secured with tape and the hind legs extended slightly caudally and positioned in a relaxed position. Sandbags or a Head End patient immobilization device may be used to support the patient's shoulders, preventing the body from tilting side to side. The sternum should be superimposed over the thoracic spine. Angle the x-ray tube 30 degrees cranially through the sacrum. Collimate the field of view to include the pelvis. See "Ventrodorsal View" under "LS Spine."

Caudal Spine

The routine views for caudal spine are VD and lateral views.

Sedation: Recommended.

Center Point: Area of interest.

Measurement Point: Proximal tail.

View: Lateral View

Place the patient in a lateral recumbent position with the fore and hind legs moderately extended cranially and caudally, respectively. Place a foam positioning wedge beneath the sternum to ensure the spine is positioned in a true lateral projection. The spine and sternum should be parallel to each other. Another foam positioning wedge may be needed beneath the abdomen to reduce obliquity of the lumbar vertebrae. The tuber ischii should be superimposed. Place the tail on thin flat radiolucent foam to keep the tail in true lateral and parallel to the tabletop. Collimate to include the area of interest (Figs. 11.30 and 11.31).

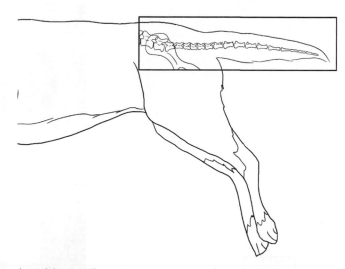

Figure 11.30.   Lateral caudal spine illustration.

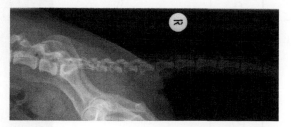

Figure 11.31.   Lateral caudal spine.

View: Ventrodorsal View

Place the patient in a dorsal recumbent position with the forelegs extended cranially and secured with tape and the hind legs extended slightly caudally and positioned in a relaxed position. Sandbags or a Head End patient immobilization device may be used to support the patient's shoulders, preventing the body from tilting side to side. The sternum should be superimposed over the thoracic spine. Collimate the field of view to include the sacrum and caudal spine (Figs. 11.32 and 11.33).

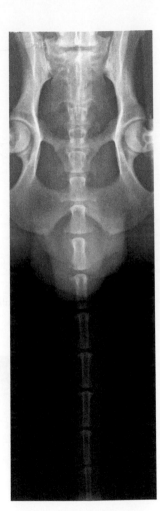

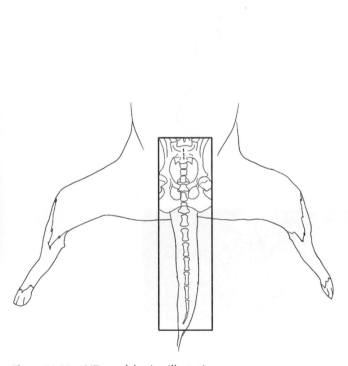

Figure 11.32.   VD caudal spine illustration.

Figure 11.33.   VD caudal spine.

Small Animal Positioning—
Thorax, Soft Tissue Neck,
and Abdomen

Thorax

The routine views for thorax imaging are dorsoventral (DV), ventrodorsal (VD), and lateral views. For evaluating the heart, DV and right lateral views are generally taken. If looking for metastatic nodules, VD and both laterals are taken. Often views chosen are clinician preference. If a patient is in respiratory distress, a DV view is taken instead of a VD. If a diaphragmatic hernia is suspected, a lateral view is taken first for the clinician to review prior to placing the patient in a VD position. A higher kVp and low mAs technique is used to attain a long scale of contrast for visualizing structures in the thorax and neck.

Sedation: None.

Center Point: Caudal dorsal border of the scapula.

Measurement Point: Highest point of the ribs.

View: Lateral View

Place the patient in lateral recumbent position, forelegs extended cranially. Place foam wedge beneath sternum so thoracic spine and sternum are parallel to each other and equidistant from the tabletop. The patient's head should be extended in a neutral position. If the head is extended too far dorsally, the image may falsely indicate a narrowing of the airway. Center over the caudal dorsal border of the scapula. Please note the forelegs should be extended before centering over the caudal dorsal border of the scapula. View is taken on inspiration (Figs. 12.1 and 12.2).

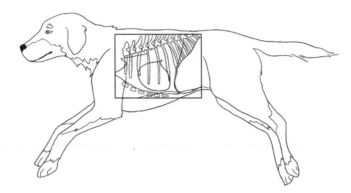

Figure 12.1.   Lateral thorax illustration.

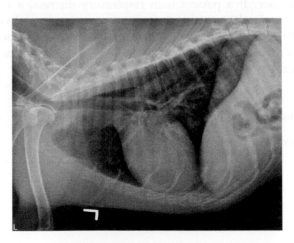

Figure 12.2.   Lateral thorax.

View: Dorsoventral View

Place patient in a sternal recumbent position with the legs extended forward and the head down on the tabletop. The sternum and spine should be superimposed and the view taken on inspiration (Figs. 12.3 and 12.4).

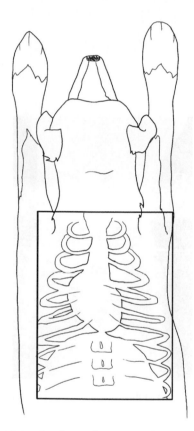

Figure 12.3. DV thorax illustration.

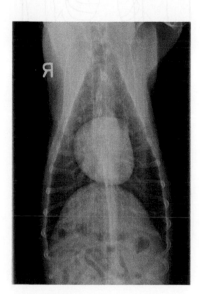

Figure 12.4. DV thorax.

View: Ventrodorsal View

Place patient in a dorsal recumbent position with the legs extended forward and the head down on the tabletop. The sternum and spine should be superimposed and the view taken on inspiration (Figs. 12.5 and 12.6).

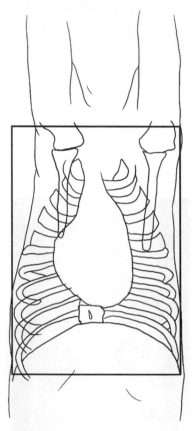

Figure 12.5. VD thorax illustration.

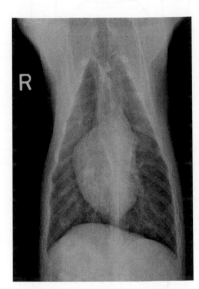

Figure 12.6. VD thorax.

Soft Tissue Neck

The routine view for imaging the soft tissue neck is a lateral view. The field of view should include the temporomandibular joints (TMJs) through the thoracic inlet. A higher kVp and low mAs technique is needed to provide a long scale of contrast. If doing the soft tissue neck in conjunction with the thorax, the same technique used for a lateral thorax can be used for the soft tissue neck.

Sedation: No.

Center Point: Mid-cervical.

Measurement Point: Shoulder area.

View: Lateral View

Place the patient in a lateral recumbent position with the head extended. The position of the head affects the obliquity of the spine. Place a wedge beneath the nose, and if the mid-cervical area appears to be sagging, place a flat piece of positioning foam to keep the spine parallel to the tabletop. The forelimbs should be extended caudally toward the abdomen. Collimate to include the area from TMJs to the thoracic inlet (Figs. 12.7 and 12.8).

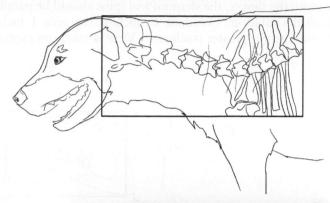

Figure 12.7. Lateral ST neck illustration.

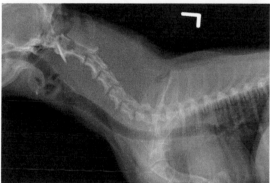

Figure 12.8. Lateral ST neck.

Abdomen

The routine views of the abdomen are VD and left or right lateral abdomen. Views chosen are often clinician preference. Supplemental views are DV, right or left lateral, flexed leg lateral, and oblique views of the abdomen. These views are taken in conjunction with special contrast enhanced procedures such as GI tract and urinary tract studies. The views are taken on expiration. For abdominal imaging, a short scale of contrast is needed to visualize abnormalities in the abdomen, so a kVp range between 50 and 90 is preferred.

Sedation: None.

Center Point: Cranial border of the abdomen should be 1 inch cranial to the tip of the xiphoid of the sternum and the caudal border should be the greater trochanter.

Measurement Point: Lateral View: Highest point of the ribs laterally.

Measurement Point: VD View: 1 inch caudal to the tip of the xiphoid of the sternum.

View: Lateral View

Place patient in lateral recumbent position with the forelegs extended cranially and the hind legs slightly extended caudally. Overextension of the hind legs can tighten the abdominal wall and compress the abdominal viscera, making interpretation more difficult. A positioning wedge should be placed beneath the sternum and an additional foam positioning wedge may be needed for the abdomen to ensure the patient is in a true lateral position. As with the thorax, the sternum and spine should be parallel to each other and equidistant from the tabletop. Collimate to include the area 1 inch cranial to the xiphoid of the sternum to the greater trochanter. View is taken on expiration (Figs. 12.9 and 12.10).

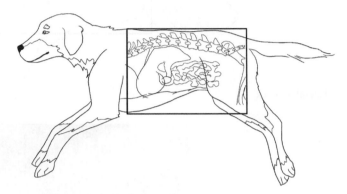

Figure 12.9.   Lateral abdomen illustration.

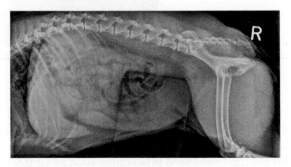

Figure 12.10.   Lateral abdomen.

View: Flexed Leg Lateral

Place patient in lateral recumbent position with the forelegs extended cranially and the hind legs placed in a neutral position. A positioning wedge should be placed beneath the sternum to ensure the patient is in a true lateral position. As with the thorax, the sternum and spine should be parallel to each other and equidistant from the tabletop. The hind legs are hyperextended cranially toward the abdomen to allow visualization of the urethra. Collimate to include the caudal abdomen in the field of view. View is taken on expiration (Figs. 12.11 and 12.12).

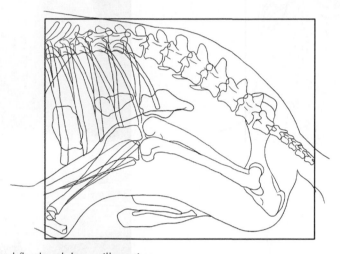

Figure 12.11. Lateral flex leg abdomen illustration.

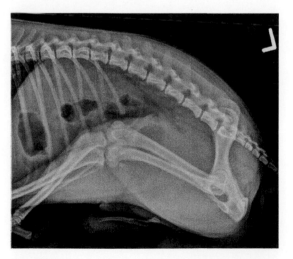

Figure 12.12. Lateral flex leg abdomen.

CHAPTER 12

View: Ventrodorsal View

Place patient in a dorsal recumbent position with the legs extended forward. The sternum and spine should be superimposed. Collimate to include the area 1 inch cranial to the xiphoid of the sternum to the greater trochanter. View is taken on expiration (Figs. 12.13 and 12.14).

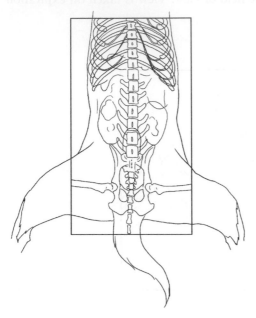

Figure 12.13.   VD abdomen illustration.

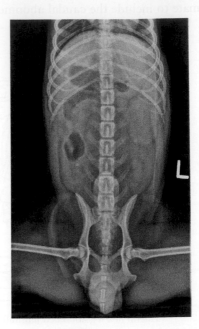

Figure 12.14.   VD abdomen.

Small Animal Positioning—Skull

For imaging of the head, care must be taken to properly place the anatomic lead markers in the field of view. The area of interest should be well collimated and if the anatomic part measures 10 cm or less, the small focal spot should be used to maximize the detail in the image. Sedation or general anesthesia is preferred for most of the imaging studies for the head.

Cranium

Routine views of the cranium are dorosoventral (DV) and lateral. Supplemental view is the frontoccipital view for the foramen magnum.

Sedation: Recommend heavy sedation or general anesthesia.

Center Point: Lateral canthus of the eye.

Measurement Point: Zygomatic arch.

View: Dorsoventral View

Place the patient in a sternal recumbent position with the forelimbs moved out of the field of view. The collimator light crosshair should be on midline and the patient's eyes should be parallel to each other. It may be necessary to use gauze or positioning foam to straighten the skull so it is not rotated. Collimate the field of view to include the whole head. The lead anatomic marker should be either on the left or right of the nose (Figs. 13.1 and 13.2).

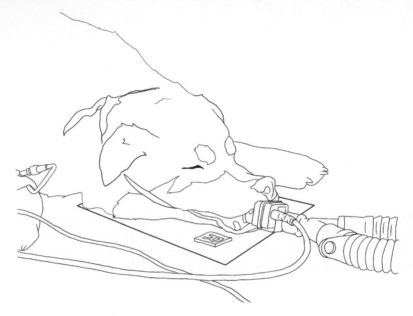

Figure 13.1.   DV cranium illustration.

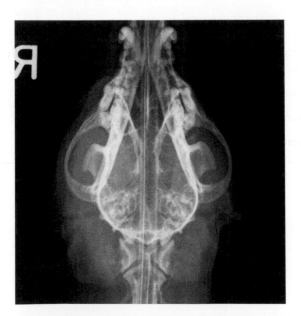

Figure 13.2.   DV cranium.

View: Lateral View

Place the patient in a lateral recumbent view with the forelegs extended caudally, out of the field of view. Place a foam positioning wedge beneath the mandible to adjust the head so it is in a true lateral position. Collimate the field of view to include the whole head. The right or left lead anatomic marker should be placed in the field of view dorsal to the maxilla or ventral to the mandible but not in the anatomy (Figs. 13.3 and 13.4).

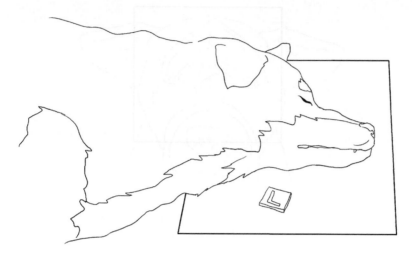

Figure 13.3.   Lateral cranium illustration.

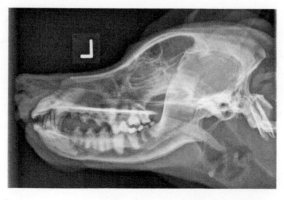

Figure 13.4.   Lateral cranium.

CHAPTER 13

View: Frontoccipital View

Place the patient in a dorsal recumbent position with the nose pointing upward and the forelegs pulled caudally toward the abdomen. Place sandbags or Head End patient immobilization device adjacent to each shoulder to support the patient. Using masking tape, tip the nose caudally approximately 30 degrees and secure by taping to the table or the immobilization device used. The patient's nose will be on his chest. Center the x-ray beam between the eyes. Collimate the field of view to include the cranium (Figs. 13.5 and 13.6).

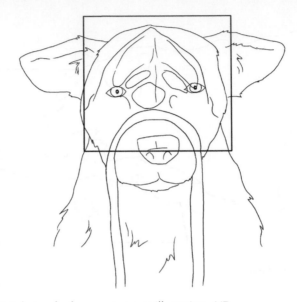

Figure 13.5.   Frontoccipital view for foramen magnum illustration—VD.

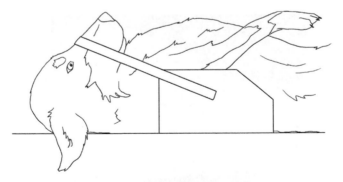

Figure 13.6.   Frontoccipital view for foramen magnum illustration—side.

Nasal

Sedation: Mandatory heavy sedation or general anesthesia.

Center Point: Lateral canthus of the eye.

Measurement Point: Zygomatic arch.

View: *Open Mouth Lateral View*

Place the patient in a lateral recumbent view with the forelegs extended caudally, out of the field of view. Place a foam positioning wedge beneath the mandible to adjust the head so it is in a true lateral position. Place a radiolucent speculum or a roll of gauze between the teeth to open the mouth. If the patient is under general anesthesia, the endotracheal tube (ET) should be tied to the mandible. Collimate the field of view to include the whole head. The right or left lead anatomic marker should be placed in the field of view dorsal to the maxilla but not in the anatomy (Figs. 13.7 and 13.8).

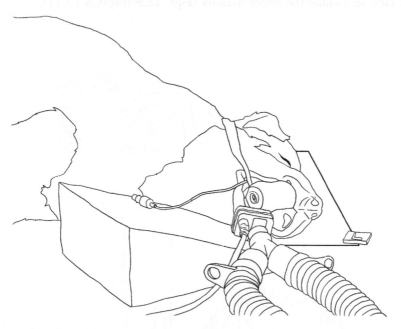

Figure 13.7. OM lateral nasal illustration.

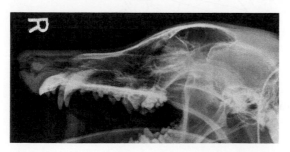

Figure 13.8. Lateral OM nasal.

View: VD Open Mouth View

Place the patient in a dorsal recumbent position with the forelegs extended caudally. Sandbags or Head End patient immobilization device should be placed against the shoulders to support the patient's body. The maxilla should be parallel to the tabletop or film cassette. Tie the ET to the mandible with the tongue beneath the ET, if under general anesthesia. Tape the maxilla to the table or cassette so it is as parallel as possible to the tabletop or cassette. Tape the mandible to the positioning device. Angle the x-ray tube 10–20 degrees caudally toward the hard palate. Note: Feline patients rarely require any x-ray tube angulation due to the range of motion when opening their mouth. Collimate the field of view to include the entire maxilla (Figs. 13.9 through 13.11).

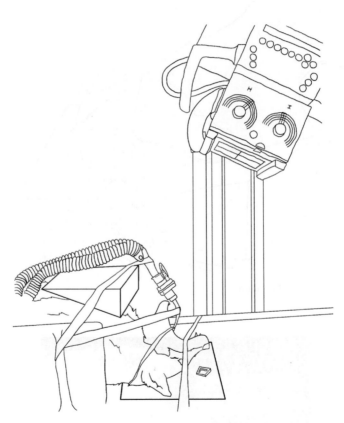

Figure 13.9.   OM soft palate side view illustration.

View: VD Frontal Sinus View

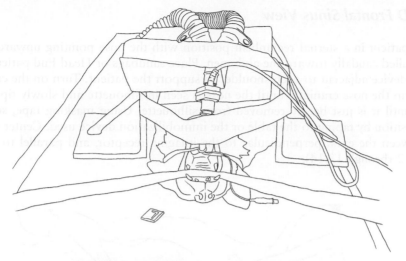

Figure 13.10.   OM soft palate cranial view illustration.

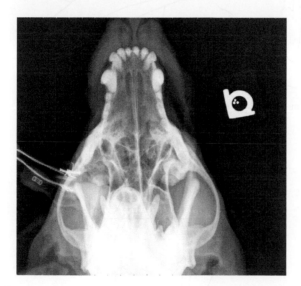

Figure 13.11.   Soft palate.

View: VD Frontal Sinus View

Place the patient in a sternal recumbent position with the nose pointing upward and the forelegs pulled caudally toward the abdomen. Place sandbags or Head End patient immobilization device adjacent to each shoulder to support the patient. Turn on the collimator light and tip the nose cranially until the nose is seen in silhouette and slowly tip the nose caudally until it is just barely removed from silhouette. Using masking tape, secure the nose in position by taping to the table or the immobilization device used. Center the x-ray beam between the eyes, perpendicular to the imaging receptor, and parallel to the nose (Figs. 13.12 through 13.14).

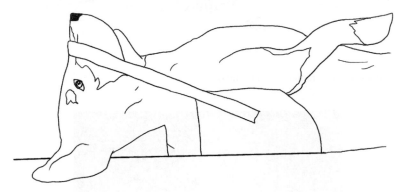

Figure 13.12.   Frontal sinus side view illustration.

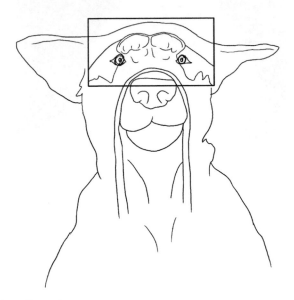

Figure 13.13.   Frontal sinus illustration.

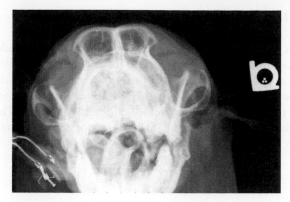

Figure 13.14. Frontal sinus.

Maxilla

The routine views of the maxilla are lateral, open mouth VD, and lateral obliques. Supplemental view may be an intra-oral view of the maxilla.

Sedation: Mandatory heavy sedation or general anesthesia.

Center Point: Lateral canthus of the eye.

Measurement Point: Zygomatic arch.

View: Open Mouth Lateral View

Place the patient in a lateral recumbent view with the forelegs extended caudally, out of the field of view. Place a foam positioning wedge beneath the mandible to adjust the head so it is in a true lateral position. Place a radiolucent speculum or a roll of gauze between the teeth to open the mouth. If under general anesthesia, the ET should be tied to the mandible. Collimate the field of view to include all of the maxilla. The right or left lead anatomic marker should be placed in the field of view dorsal to the maxilla but not in the anatomy (Figs. 13.15 and 13.16).

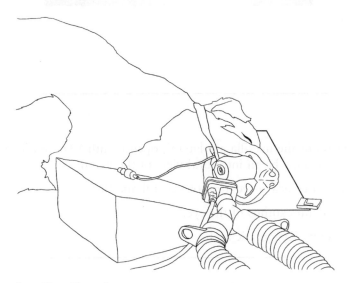

Figure 13.15.   Lateral maxillary illustration.

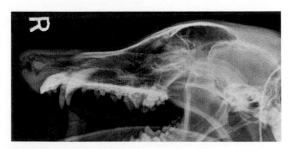

Figure 13.16.   Lateral maxillary.

View: VD Open Mouth View

Place the patient in a dorsal recumbent position with the forelegs extended caudally. Sandbags or Head End patient immobilization device should be placed against the shoulders to support the patient's body. The maxilla should be parallel to the tabletop or film cassette. Tie the ET to the mandible with the tongue beneath the ET, if under general anesthesia. Tape the maxilla to the table or cassette so it is as parallel as possible to the tabletop or cassette. Tape the mandible to the positioning device. Angle the x-ray tube 10–20 degrees caudally toward the hard palate. Note: Feline patients rarely require any x-ray tube angulation due to the range of motion when opening their mouth. Collimate the field of view to include the entire maxilla (Figs. 13.17 and 13.18).

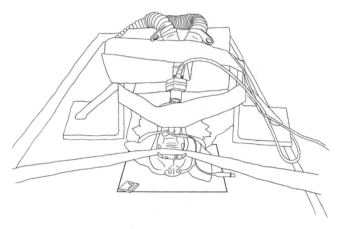

Figure 13.17.   Soft palate illustration.

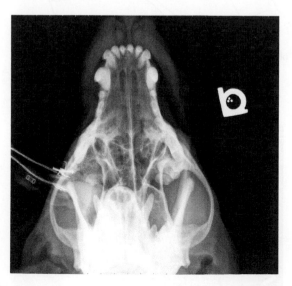

Figure 13.18.   Soft palate.

View: Open Mouth Oblique View—Upper Dental Arcade

Place the patient in a lateral recumbent position with the forelegs extended caudally. If the patient is under general anesthesia, tie the ET to the mandible. Place a radiolucent speculum in the patient's mouth. Rotate the body halfway dorsally and place a foam positioning wedge beneath the mandible. Rotate the head approximately 45 degrees from lateral so there is not superimposition from the opposite maxillary arcade. The arcade visualized is the one closest to the cassette or tabletop. The right and left anatomic lead markers should be placed dorsal and ventral to the maxilla. Note: It is helpful to collimate out part of the mandibular arcade so there is no confusion regarding which arcade is being imaged. Do not place the right and left markers dorsal to the maxilla and ventral to the mandible (Figs. 13.19 and 13.20).

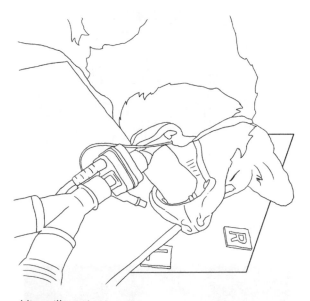

Figure 13.19.   Maxillary oblique illustration.

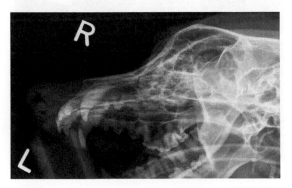

Figure 13.20.   Maxillary oblique.

Mandible

The routine views of the mandible are lateral, DV, and lateral oblique views. An intraoral view may be requested for rostral mandibular fractures or disease. With DR, a conventional intraoral view may not be possible. An open mouth angled projection will show the mandibular symphysis, though not as well as the intraoral view.

Sedation: Mandatory heavy sedation or general anesthesia.

Center Point: Lateral canthus of the eye.

Measurement Point: Zygomatic arch.

View: Lateral Open Mouth

Place the patient in a lateral recumbent view with the forelegs extended caudally, out of the field of view. Place a foam positioning wedge beneath the mandible to adjust the head so it is in a true lateral position. Place a radiolucent speculum or a roll of gauze between the teeth to open the mouth. If under general anesthesia, the ET should be tied to the maxilla. Collimate the field of view to include all of the mandible. The right or left lead anatomic marker should be placed in the field of view ventral to the mandible but not in the anatomy (Figs. 13.21 and 13.22).

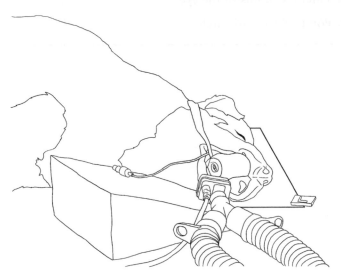

Figure 13.21.   Lateral mandible illustration.

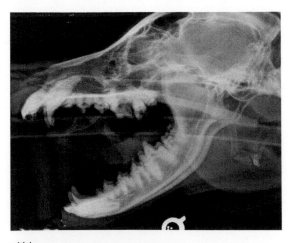

Figure 13.22.   Lateral mandible.

View: Dorsoventral View

Place the patient in a sternal recumbent position with the forelimbs moved out of the field of view. The collimator light crosshair should be on midline and the patient's eyes should be parallel to each other. It may be necessary to use gauze or positioning foam to straighten the skull so it is not rotated. Collimate the field of view to include the mandible. The lead anatomic marker should be either on the left or right of the nose (Figs. 13.23 and 13.24).

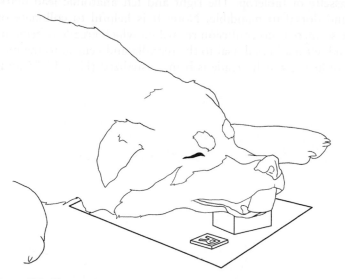

Figure 13.23.   DV mandible illustration.

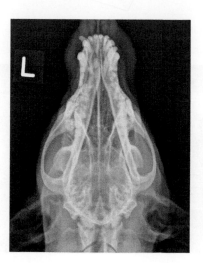

Figure 13.24.   DV mandible.

View: Lateral Oblique Open Mouth

Place the patient in a lateral recumbent position with the forelegs extended caudally. If the patient is under general anesthesia, tie the ET to the maxilla. Place a radiolucent speculum in the patient's mouth. Place a foam positioning wedge behind the skull so the head is rotated approximately 20–30 degrees. The angle chosen is dependent upon the shape of the dog's head. A brachycephalic breed may only need 20 degrees obliquity, whereas a dolichocephalic or mesaticephalic breed may need 30 degrees. The goal is to minimize any superimposition from the opposite mandibular arcade. The arcade visualized is the one closest to the cassette or tabletop. The right and left anatomic lead markers should be placed ventral and dorsal to mandible. Note: It is helpful to collimate out part of the maxillary arcade so there is no confusion regarding which arcade is being imaged. Do not place the right and left markers dorsal to the maxilla and ventral to the mandible because it may become confusing which arcade is being visualized (Figs. 13.25 and 13.26).

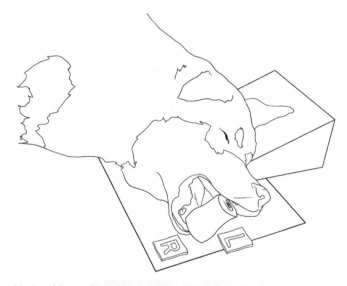

Figure 13.25.   Mandibular oblique illustration.

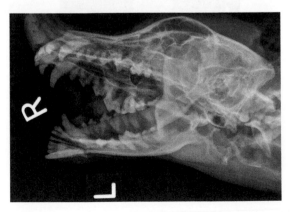

Figure 13.26.   Mandibular oblique.

View: Modified Mandibular Symphysis Projection for DR

Place the patient in a sternal recumbent position with the forelimbs moved out of the field of view. The patient's rostral mandible should be placed on a small foam positioning block or on a stack of gauze to ensure the mandible is parallel to the tabletop. Roll gauze should be placed in the patient's mouth as caudal as possible to open the mouth as wide as possible. The collimator light crosshair should be on midline and angled approximately 15 degrees caudally to be centered on the mandibular symphysis. The patient's eyes should be parallel to each other. It may be necessary to use gauze or positioning foam to straighten the skull so it is not rotated. Collimate to include as much of the rostral mandible as possible. The lead anatomic marker should be either on the left or right of the mandible (Figs. 13.27 and 13.28).

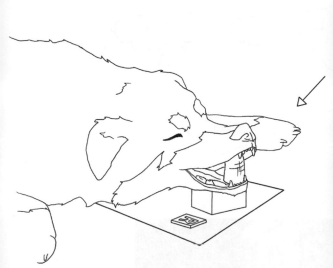

Figure 13.27. OM view mandibular symphysis illustration—DR; arrow demonstrates x-ray tube angle.

Figure 13.28. OM view mandibular symphysis—DR.

CHAPTER 13

Temporomandibular Joints

The routine views for imaging temporomandibular joints (TMJs) are DV closed mouth, lateral craniocaudal oblique mouth and open and closed with the nose tipped up 20 degrees, and an open mouth basilar view.

Sedation: Heavy sedation or general anesthesia.

Center Point: TMJ.

Measurement Point: TMJ.

View: Dorsoventral Closed Mouth View

Place the patient in a sternal recumbent position with the forelimbs moved out of the field of view. The collimator light crosshair should be on midline and the patient's eyes should be parallel to each other. It may be necessary to use gauze or positioning foam to straighten the skull so it is not rotated. Collimate the field of view to include the mandible. The lead anatomic marker should be either on the left or right of the nose (Figs. 13.29 and 13.30).

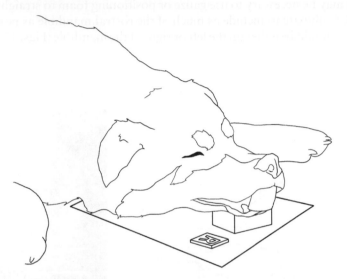

Figure 13.29.   DV TMJ illustration.

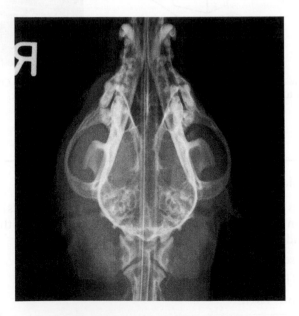

Figure 13.30.   DV TMJ.

View: *Basilar or Ventrodorsal Open Mouth View*

Place the patient in a dorsal recumbent position with the patient's nose directed upward and the mouth opened by using either gauze or masking tape to pull the maxillary arcade slightly cranial and the mandible caudally. The corners of the mouth should be positioned over C2. The forelegs are pulled caudally and secured with tape. The patient should be in a true VD position with the sternum and spine superimposed and the cervical spine parallel to the tabletop. The ET should be removed or tied to the mandible. Center over the commissure of the lips (Figs. 13.31 and 13.32).

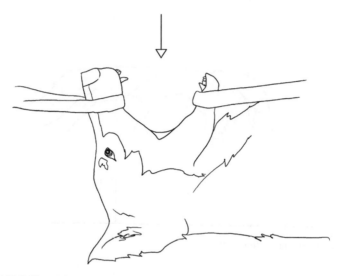

Figure 13.31. OM TMJ illustration.

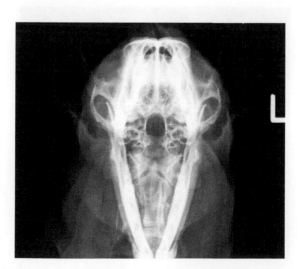

Figure 13.32. OM VD TMJ.

View: Lateral Craniocaudal Oblique of the Mouth, Open and Closed

Place the patient in a lateral recumbent position with the affected side down. Tip the nose up and place a 20-degree wedge beneath the rostral mandible to elevate the mandible and rotate the cranium slightly toward the tabletop. The degree of angulation is contingent upon the shape of the patient's head. Make exposures with the mouth closed and open bilaterally. The anatomic lead marker should denote the TMJ being visualized and should be placed ventral to the TMJ (Figs. 13.33 and 13.34).

If the mouth cannot be opened or the ET is overlying the TM joint, place patient in a true lateral position and tip the nose up 20 degrees so the down TMJ is projected forward (Figs. 13.35 and 13.36).

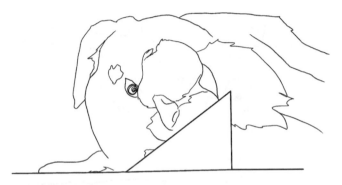

Figure 13.33.   Lateral oblique illustration TMJ.

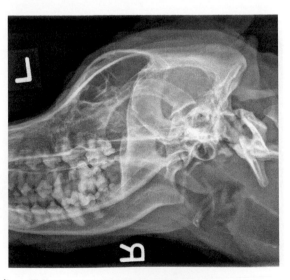

Figure 13.34.   Lateral oblique TMJ.

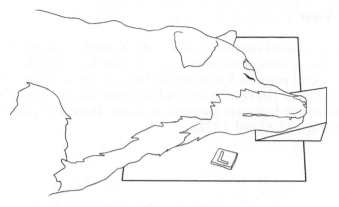

Figure 13.35.   Lateral 20-degree nose up illustration.

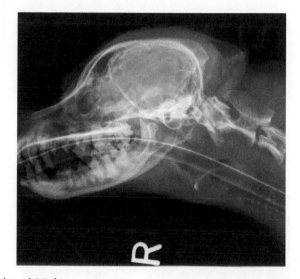

Figure 13.36.   Straight lateral 20-degree nose up.

Tympanic Bullae

The routine views for imaging canine tympanic bullae are lateral, DV with the mouth closed, lateral craniocaudal oblique with the mouth closed, and basilar or ventrodorsal open mouth views. The routine views for imaging feline tympanic bullae are lateral, DV with the mouth closed, lateral craniocaudal oblique with the mouth closed, and basilar or ventrodorsal open mouth or ventrodorsal closed mouth views.

Sedation: Heavy sedation or general anesthesia.

Center Point: Bullae.

Measurement Point: Bullae.

View: Lateral View

Place the patient in a lateral recumbent view with the forelegs extended caudally, out of the field of view. Place a foam positioning wedge beneath the mandible to adjust the head so it is in a true lateral position. Collimate the field of view to include from the lateral canthus of the eye to C2. The right or left lead anatomic marker should be placed in the field of view ventral to the bullae but not in the anatomy. There is no change when imaging the feline patient (Figs. 13.37 and 13.38).

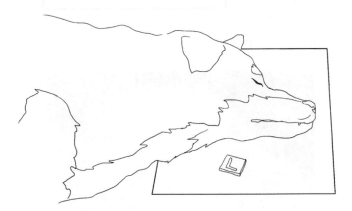

Figure 13.37.   Lateral bullae illustration.

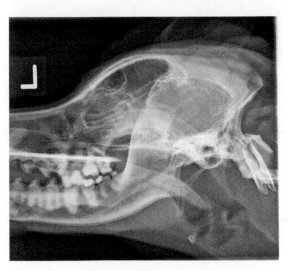

Figure 13.38.   Lateral bullae.

View: *Dorsoventral View*

Place the patient in a sternal recumbent position with the forelimbs moved out of the field of view. The collimator light crosshair should be on midline and the patient's eyes should be parallel to each other. It may be necessary to use gauze or positioning foam to straighten the skull so it is not rotated. Center over the bullae and collimate the field of view to include the lateral canthus to C2. The lead anatomic marker should be either on the left or right of the cranium. There is no change when imaging the feline patient (Figs. 13.39 and 13.40).

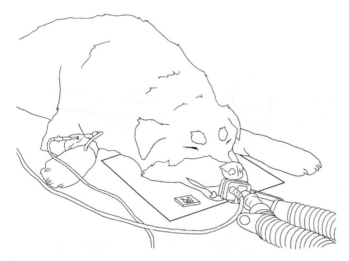

Figure 13.39.   DV bullae illustration.

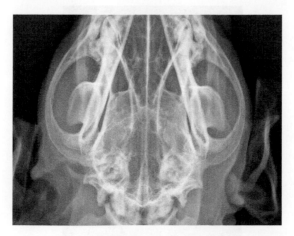

Figure 13.40.   DV bullae.

View: Basilar or Ventrodorsal Open Mouth View

Place the patient in a dorsal recumbent position with the patient's nose directed upward and the mouth opened by using either gauze or masking tape to pull the maxillary arcade slightly cranial and the mandible caudally. The commissure of the lips should be positioned over the bullae. The forelegs are pulled caudally and secured with tape. The patient should be in a true VD position with the sternum and spine superimposed and the cervical spine parallel to the tabletop. The ET should be removed or tied to the mandible. Center over the commissure of the lips. There is no change when imaging the feline patient (Figs. 13.41 and 13.42).

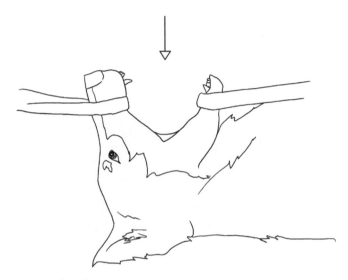

Figure 13.41.   OM canine bullae illustration.

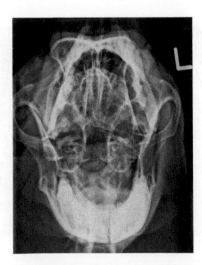

Figure 13.42.   OM canine bullae.

View: Lateral Craniocaudal Oblique View with Mouth Closed

Place the patient in a lateral recumbent position with the forelegs extended caudally. The unaffected tympanic bullae should be toward the tabletop. Place a foam positioning wedge behind the skull so the head is rotated approximately 20 degrees to separate the bullae. The nose should be tipped cranially to prevent TMJ superimposition. The right and left anatomic lead markers should be placed ventral and dorsal to cranium near the bullae. The feline patient does not require a foam positioning wedge to be placed behind the cranium for the oblique views. The feline cranium will naturally tilt approximately 10 degrees, which will separate the tympanic bullae. The nose should be tipped cranially to prevent TMJ superimposition as with the canine patient (Figs. 13.43 and 13.44).

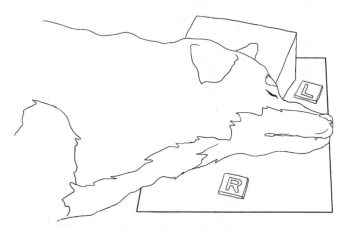

Figure 13.43.   Oblique canine bullae illustration.

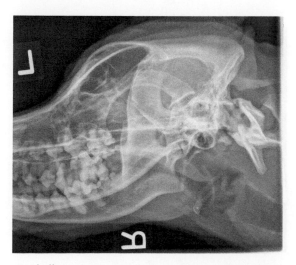

Figure 13.44.   Oblique canine bullae.

View: Feline Ventrodorsal Closed Mouth View

Place the feline patient in a dorsal recumbent position with the patient's nose directed upward and the mouth closed. Tilt the nose cranially approximately 20 degrees and center over the bullae. The forelegs are pulled caudally and secured with tape. The patient should be in a true VD position with the sternum and spine superimposed and the cervical spine parallel to the tabletop. Due to the location of the feline bullae, the bullae and often the odontoid process can be visualized with this view (Figs. 13.45 and 13.46).

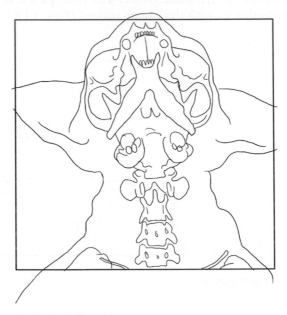

Figure 13.45.   Feline VD closed mouth illustration.

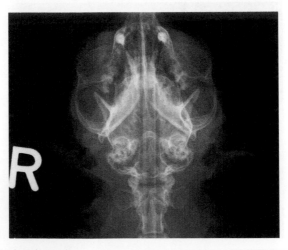

Figure 13.46.   Feline VD closed mouth.

14

Exotic Pet Imaging

Avian and exotic pets have increased in popularity, particularly within the last decade. Imaging this type of patient can be a challenge to both the patient and the radiographer. Most small exotic pets, like hamsters, guinea pigs, and rabbits, can be imaged in a similar fashion to the regular small animal patient. Imaging birds and reptiles is a little different due to the restraint needed to protect the patient as well as the radiographer. Birds, domestic or wild, are easily stressed and do not tolerate long procedures well. Reptiles, depending upon species, require special handling. The restraint method for birds is dependent upon the type and size of the patient and the imaging exam being performed. A bird board is a plexiglass positioning aid useful for both avian and some reptile patients. It is particularly helpful if the patient is a raptor, psittacine, or poisonous or more aggressive reptile. Simple supplies like masking tape, gauze rolls, leather gloves, and terrycloth towels are necessary when imaging the exotic pet. This chapter will cover basic positioning for small mammals, reptiles, and birds. In the special procedures chapter, there is additional information included for performing contrast enhanced special procedures on small mammals and birds.

Avian

The routine views for whole body views of the avian patient are ventrodorsal (VD) and lateral views. The restraint method for birds is dependent upon the type and size of the patient. Leather gloves should be worn when handling parrots and raptors. The kVp range typically used for avian imaging is 48–65 kVp. The mAs needed is dependent upon the type of image receptor being used. Film screen imaging mAs range would be 5–10 mAs. With digital imaging, 5 mAs would suffice.

Sedation: None.

Equipment: Bird board restraint device, leather gloves, masking tape, gauze rolls, and towel.

View: Ventrodorsal View

Before positioning the avian patient, the room should be set up so the patient is handled and restrained for a minimal amount of time. If imaging a parrot or raptor, leather gloves should be worn when placing the patient on the bird board. Masking tape is the best tape to use when taping the wings down on a bird. When the tape is removed, always remove it in the direction the feathers are pointed. If imaging a raptor or parrot, placing a gauze roll for each foot so the bird can grasp it will help prevent having fingers or clothes grasped by the bird. The room should be quiet and the lights slightly dimmed to reduce stress for parrots and raptors. It will take a minimum of two staff to image the avian patient, one to place and restrain the bird while the other tapes the bird to the board. Tape should be cut and ready to be placed prior to placing the bird on a commercial bird board or a piece of plexiglass. If using a commercial bird board, place the patient on the board and place the neck restraint first to secure the head. Next, secure each leg while the holder continues to protect the wings and separate the legs. With the head and legs restrained, stretch the wings out laterally and tape the wings down midway bilaterally. Lastly, place another strip of tape on the distal portion of the wings bilaterally. Place the bird board on the tabletop on a film cassette or DR panel, anatomically mark the image, and make the exposure (Figs. 14.1 through 14.3).

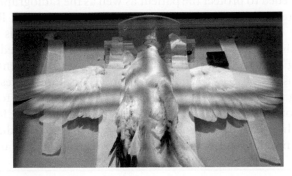

Figure 14.1.   VD dove on bird board.

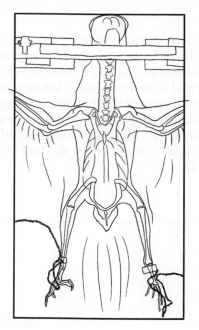

Figure 14.2. Avian VD illustration parrot.

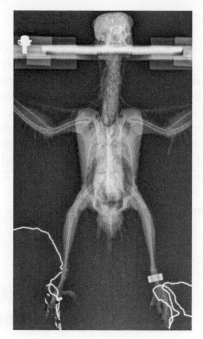

Figure 14.3. Avian VD parrot image.

View: Lateral View

To take the lateral view, release and hold the up leg, have the assisting tech untape the wings, and gently turn the patient laterally, while the tech wearing the leather gloves readjusts the head as the patient is turned. Retape and secure the leg. Extend the wings dorsally and place a thin radiolucent positioning foam pad between the wings before taping them securely back to the bird board. Take the lateral exposure. When the imaging is complete, untape the wings and move them back against the body of the bird. Untape the legs/feet and hold them in one hand gloved hand. Grasp the bird's head with the other gloved hand and have the assisting tech release the head restraint. Place the bird in its carrier and cover with a towel (Figs. 14.4 through 14.6).

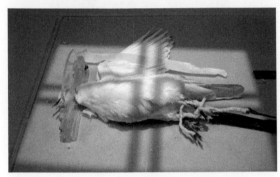

Figure 14.4.   Lateral projection dove on board.

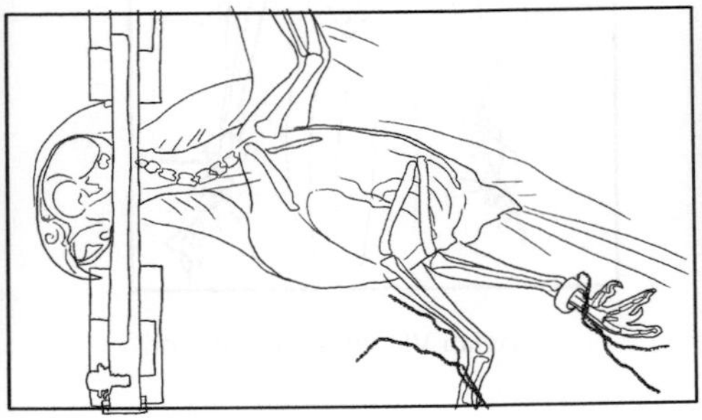

Figure 14.5.   Avian lateral illustration parrot.

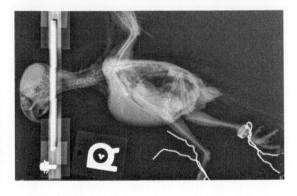

Figure 14.6.   Lateral whole body parrot.

Small Mammals

Routine views for small mammals are the same as for the canine and feline patient. Restraint techniques may vary and include physical and chemical restraint.

Sedation: Recommended.

Center Point: Same guidelines as canine and feline patients.

Measurement Point: Same guidelines as canine and feline patients.

View: *Lateral View*

Depending upon the imaging exam requested, it may be necessary to take a horizontal beam image to attain the lateral projection, particularly if the patient is not sedated. Using gauze rolls to extend extremities is a frequently used restraint method, as well as using tape. If using tape, adding a strip of tape to the adhesive side of a previously cut strip of tape, leaving only the ends of the tape uncovered, is also a technique used to tape down some small mammals (or budgies) so they do not lose hair or feathers (Figs. 14.7 and 14.8).

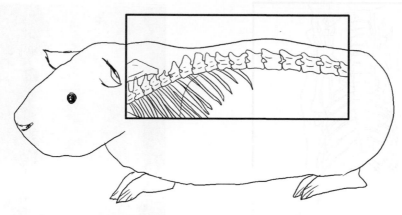

Figure 14.7.   Lateral view guinea pig illustration.

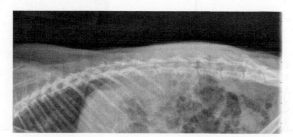

Figure 14.8.   Lateral view guinea pig spine.

View: Ventrodorsal versus Dorsoventral Views

Dorsoventral (DV) views of the thorax and abdomen are usually easier on the exotic patient than placing the animal in a dorsal recumbent position. Restraining an unsedated small mammal, like a hamster or gerbil, can be attained by placing it in a plexiglass box or a toilet paper roll with the ends covered. Rabbits are susceptible to spinal injuries, so care should be taken if imaging an unsedated rabbit (Figs. 14.9 and 14.10).

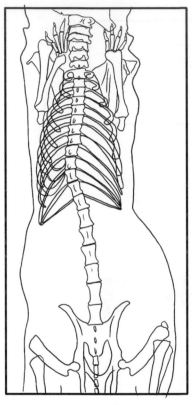

Figure 14.9.   VD guinea pig illustration.

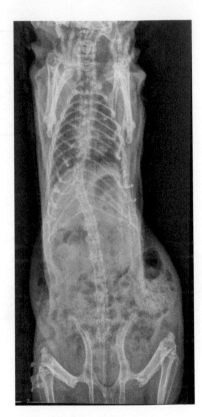

Figure 14.10.   VD guinea pig spine.

Reptile

Routine views for reptiles are the same as for the canine and feline patient. Restraint techniques may vary and include physical and chemical restraint.

Sedation: Recommended.

Center Point: Same guidelines as canine and feline patients.

Measurement Point: Same guidelines as canine and feline patients.

View: Lateral View

Depending upon the imaging exam requested, it may be necessary to take a horizontal beam image to attain the lateral projection, particularly if the patient is not sedated (Figs. 14.11 through 14.13).

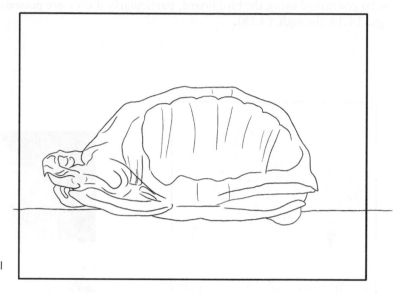

Figure 14.11. X table lateral view turtle illustration.

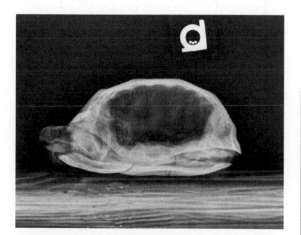

Figure 14.12. X table lateral turtle image.

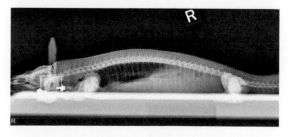

Figure 14.13. X table gila monster on board.

View: Ventrodorsal versus Dorsoventral Views

DV views of the thorax and abdomen are usually easier on the exotic patient than placing it in a dorsal recumbent position. Restraining an unsedated reptile can be attained by placing the reptile in a plexiglass box, or if imaging a snake, place it in a bag. Some reptiles can be restrained using the bird board, particularly if they are poisonous and/or aggressive (Figs. 14.14 through 14.18).

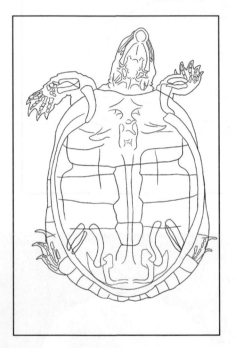

Figure 14.14.   DV turtle illustration.

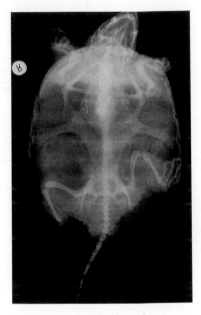

Figure 14.15.   DV whole body turtle.

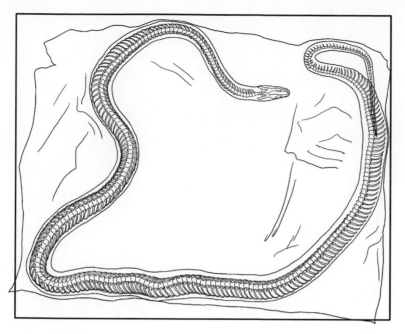

Figure 14.16.   Snake in bag illustration.

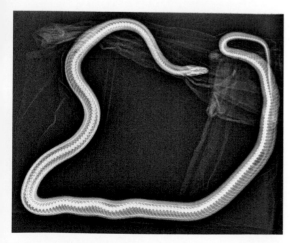

Figure 14.17.   Snake in bag image.

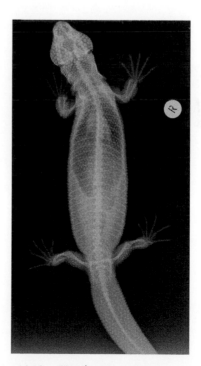

Figure 14.18.   DV gila monster image.

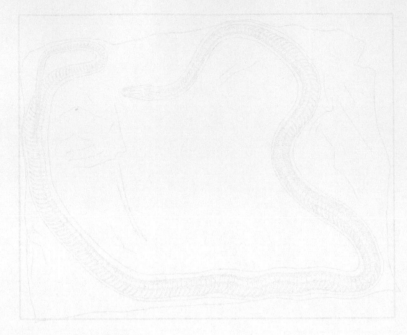

Snake in bag illustration.

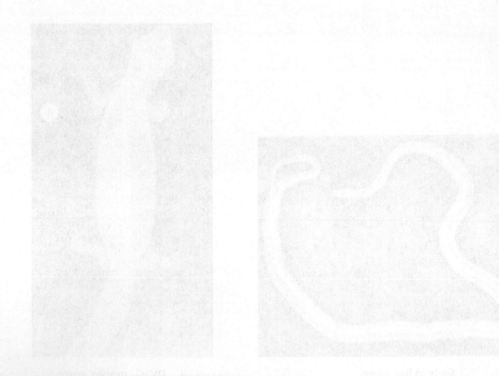

Section 3

Contrast Media and Special Procedures

Radiopaque Contrast Media

Special contrast enhanced imaging procedures are performed to better visualize soft tissue structures or organs when survey imaging does not give the practitioner the needed information for diagnosis. The most common contrast imaging exams performed in a small animal practice are for imaging vasculature, GI tract, genitourinary tract, spinal canal (myelography), fistulae, and joints.

The basic two types of contrast enhancement used are positive and negative. Positive contrast enhancement requires the use of two common radiopaque contrast media, iodine and barium. Negative contrast enhancement requires the use of gases that have a low specific gravity (carbon dioxide or oxygen).[10] To assist the small animal practitioner and the veterinary technician, it is important to review the radiopaque contrast media (**ROCM**) types and dosage information most commonly used for the veterinary patient.

Types of Radiopaque Contrast Media

Radiopaque contrast media are high-density pharmacologic agents use to opacify low contrast tissues in the body.[13,15] Iodine and barium are the most commonly used contrast agents. They have a higher atomic number and mass density than the low contrast tissues of the body and absorb more x-rays than soft tissue or bone[13] (Fig. 15.1).

Ionic and Nonionic Contrast Agents

Water-soluble iodine agents are either ionic or nonionic. The first organic iodine-based contrast agent was produced in the 1930s, and tri-iodinated compounds became available in the 1950s. Diatrizoate, metrizoate, and iothalmate are three of the most

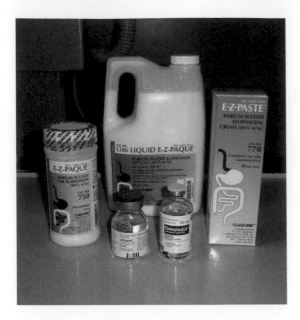

Figure 15.1. Contrast media types.

common tri-iodinated compounds. Tri-iodinated compounds contain three atoms of iodine per molecule. In the 1960s, it was determined that many of the adverse effects of iodinated contrast media were due to their hypertonicity. Basically, ionic contrast agents have an osmolality between 1,900 and 2,100 mOsm/kg water while blood has osmolality of 290 and 900 mOsm/kg water, depending upon the contrast agent. Osmolality is the number of milliosmoles per kilogram of water or the concentration of molecules per weight of water. When highly osmotic substances, such as ionic radiopaque contrast media, are placed in the bloodstream, fluid from outside of the bloodstream (extravascular space) will be drawn into the bloodstream (intravascular space). This dilutes the osmotic particles until osmotic pressures balance between the intravascular and extravascular spaces, increasing the intravascular hydrostatic (fluid) pressures. Ionic contrast media is hypertonic to plasma at the concentrations needed for imaging.

Nonionic contrast agents have an osmolality closer to blood in a range between 290 and 900 mOsm/kg water, depending upon the contrast agent used. The nonionic low-osmolar monomer compounds have an estimated one-third the osmolality of conventional ionic iodine salts at the same iodine concentration. Fewer side effects permit more concentrated and greater volumes of contrast to be used when needed to improve visualization of a structure or region. There is less patient motion due to the reduced side effects and increased patient comfort. Also, the nonionic contrast media agents are diluted more slowly and to a lesser extent than ionic contrast, resulting in sharper contrast borders for an increased length of time. Lastly, nonionic contrast media agents are estimated to be six times safer than ionic contrast media due to nonionicity and the reduction in hypertonicity, chemical toxicity, and allergic reactions.[13,14] They are a little more expensive but they have decreased in cost in recent years. Care must be taken when preparing the contrast media dose for some special imaging procedures like myelography. If myelographic exams are performed in the practice rarely or routinely, it may be useful to have a myelographic dose table available for quick reference due to the dose variation for cisternal tap versus lumbar tap when administering the contrast (Table 15.1).

Table 15.1.   Myelographic Dose Table - Omnipaque 240.

BW kg	TL Spine 0.3 ml/ kg	C Spine 0.5 ml/ kg	C Spine & Tap 0.2 ml/kg	BW kg	TL Spine 0.3 ml/ kg	C Spine 0.5 ml/ kg	C Spine &Tap 0.2 ml/kg	BW kg	TL Spine 0.3 ml/ kg	C Spine 0.5 ml/ kg	C Spine & Tap 0.2 ml/kg
0.5	0.2	0.3	0.1	20.9	6.3	10.5	4.2	41.4	12.4	20.7	8.3
0.9	0.3	0.5	0.2	21.4	6.4	10.7	4.3	41.8	12.5	20.9	8.4
1.4	0.4	0.7	0.3	21.8	6.5	10.9	4.4	42.3	12.7	21.2	8.5
1.8	0.5	0.9	0.4	22.3	6.7	11.2	4.5	42.7	12.8	21.4	8.5
2.3	0.7	1.2	0.5	22.7	6.8	11.4	4.5	43.2	13.0	21.6	8.6
2.7	0.8	1.4	0.5	23.2	7.0	11.6	4.6	43.6	13.1	21.8	8.7
3.2	1.0	1.6	0.6	23.6	7.1	11.8	4.7	44.1	13.2	22.1	8.8
3.6	1.1	1.8	0.7	24.1	7.2	12.1	4.8	44.5	13.4	22.3	8.9
4.1	1.2	2.1	0.8	24.5	7.4	12.3	4.9	45.0	13.5	22.5	9.0
4.5	1.4	2.3	0.9	25.0	7.5	12.5	5.0	45.5	13.7	22.8	9.1
5.0	1.5	2.5	1.0	25.5	7.7	12.8	5.1	45.9	13.8	23.0	9.2
5.5	1.7	2.8	1.1	25.9	7.8	13.0	5.2	46.4	13.9	23.2	9.3
5.9	1.8	3.0	1.2	26.4	7.9	13.2	5.3	46.8	14.0	23.4	9.4
6.4	1.9	3.2	1.3	26.8	8.0	13.4	5.4	47.3	14.2	23.7	9.5
6.8	2.0	3.4	1.4	27.3	8.2	13.7	5.5	47.4	14.2	23.7	9.5
7.3	2.2	3.7	1.5	27.7	8.3	13.9	5.5	48.2	14.5	24.1	9.6
7.7	2.3	3.9	1.5	28.2	8.5	14.1	5.6	48.6	14.6	24.3	9.7
8.2	2.5	4.1	1.6	28.6	8.6	14.3	5.7	49.1	14.7	24.6	9.8
8.6	2.6	4.3	1.7	29.1	8.7	14.6	5.8	49.5	14.9	24.8	9.9
9.1	2.7	4.6	1.8	29.5	8.9	14.8	5.9	50.0	15.0	25.0	10.0
9.5	2.9	4.8	1.9	30.0	9.0	15.0	6.0	50.5	15.2	25.3	10.1
10.0	3.0	5.0	2.0	30.5	9.2	15.3	6.1	50.9	15.3	25.5	10.2
10.5	3.2	5.3	2.1	30.9	9.3	15.5	6.2	51.4	15.4	25.7	10.3
10.9	3.3	5.5	2.2	31.4	9.4	15.7	6.3	51.8	15.5	25.9	10.4
11.4	3.4	5.7	2.3	31.8	9.5	15.9	6.4	52.3	15.7	26.2	10.5
11.8	3.5	5.9	2.4	32.2	9.7	16.2	6.5	52.7	15.8	26.4	10.5
12.3	3.7	6.2	2.5	32.7	9.8	16.4	6.5	53.2	16.0	26.6	10.6
12.7	3.8	6.4	2.5	33.2	10.0	16.6	6.6	53.6	16.1	26.8	10.7
13.2	4.0	6.6	2.6	33.6	10.1	16.8	6.7	54.1	16.2	27.1	10.8
13.6	4.1	6.8	2.7	34.1	10.2	17.1	6.8	54.5	16.4	27.3	10.9
14.1	4.2	7.0	2.8	34.5	10.4	17.3	6.9	55.0	16.5	27.5	11.0
14.5	4.4	7.3	2.9	35.0	10.5	17.5	7.0	55.5	16.7	27.8	11.1
15.0	4.5	7.5	3.0	35.5	10.7	17.8	7.1	55.9	16.8	28.0	11.2
15.5	4.7	7.8	3.1	35.9	10.8	18.0	7.2	56.4	16.9	28.2	11.3
15.9	4.8	8.0	3.2	36.4	10.9	18.2	7.2	56.8	17.0	28.4	11.4
16.4	4.9	8.2	3.3	36.8	11.0	18.4	7.4	57.1	17.1	28.6	11.4
16.8	5.0	8.4	3.4	37.3	11.2	18.7	7.5	57.7	17.3	28.9	11.5
17.3	5.2	8.7	3.5	37.7	11.3	18.9	7.5	58.2	17.5	29.1	11.6
17.7	5.3	8.9	3.5	38.2	11.5	19.1	7.6	58.6	17.6	29.3	11.7
18.2	5.5	9.1	3.6	38.6	11.6	19.3	7.7	59.1	17.7	29.6	11.8
18.6	5.6	9.3	3.7	39.1	11.7	19.6	7.8	59.5	17.9	29.8	11.9
19.1	5.7	9.6	3.8	39.5	11.9	19.8	7.9	60.0	18.0	30.0	12.0
19.5	5.9	9.8	3.9	40.0	12.0	20.0	8.0	60.5	18.2	30.3	12.1
20.0	6.0	10.0	4.0	40.5	12.2	20.3	8.1	60.9	18.3	30.5	12.2
20.5	6.2	10.3	4.1	40.9	12.3	20.5	8.2	61.4	18.4	30.7	12.3

Table 15.2.   Body Weight Conversion Table.

lb	kg	lb	kg	lb	kg	lb	kg
1	0.5	39	17.7	77	35.0	115	52.3
2	0.9	40	18.2	78	35.5	116	52.7
3	1.4	41	18.6	79	35.9	117	53.2
4	1.8	42	19.1	80	36.4	118	53.6
5	2.3	43	19.5	81	36.8	119	54.1
6	2.7	44	20.0	82	37.3	120	54.5
7	3.2	45	20.5	83	37.7	121	55.0
8	3.6	46	20.9	84	38.2	122	55.5
9	4.1	47	21.4	85	38.6	123	55.9
10	4.5	48	21.8	86	39.1	124	56.4
11	5.0	49	22.3	87	39.5	125	56.8
12	5.5	50	22.7	88	40.0	126	59.1
13	5.9	51	23.2	89	40.5	127	57.7
14	6.4	52	23.6	90	40.9	128	58.2
15	6.8	53	24.1	91	41.4	129	58.6
16	7.3	54	24.5	92	41.8	130	59.1
17	7.7	55	25.0	93	42.3	131	59.5
18	8.2	56	25.5	94	42.7	132	60.0
19	8.6	57	25.9	95	43.2	133	60.5
20	9.1	58	26.4	96	43.6	134	60.9
21	9.5	59	26.8	97	44.1	135	61.4
22	10.0	60	27.3	98	44.5	136	61.8
23	10.5	61	27.7	99	45.0	137	62.3
24	10.9	62	28.2	100	45.5	138	62.7
25	11.4	63	28.6	101	45.9	139	63.2
26	11.8	64	29.1	102	46.4	140	63.6
27	12.3	65	29.5	103	46.8	141	64.1
28	12.7	66	30.0	104	47.3	142	64.5
29	13.2	67	30.5	105	47.4	143	65.0
30	13.6	68	30.9	106	48.2	144	65.5
31	14.1	69	31.4	107	48.6	145	65.9
32	14.5	70	31.8	108	49.1	146	66.4
33	15.0	71	32.2	109	49.5	147	66.8
34	15.5	72	32.7	110	50.0	148	67.3
35	15.9	73	33.2	111	50.5	149	67.7
36	16.4	74	33.6	112	50.9	150	68.2
37	16.8	75	34.1	113	51.4		
38	17.3	76	34.5	114	51.8		

Another handy reference table to have available when preparing contrast media doses is a body weight conversion table (Table 15.2).

Allergic reactions and side effects to contrast agents are not as common in the veterinary patient as in humans, but they do happen. It is extremely important to make sure a patient is well hydrated before performing any contrast procedure. When using ionic contrast media agents, systemic reactions can occur acutely or be delayed. Most reactions occur within the first 5–10 minutes post-administration and range from mild to fatal. There is no way to determine how severe a reaction will be. Ionic contrast media agents are more anti-coagulant than nonionic media and are less likely to develop clot formation in the catheter or syringe. The types of side effects and reactions can range from but are not limited to acute renal failure (which can be dose-dependent), ECG changes, respiratory arrest, peripheral vasodilatation, nausea, and vomiting. The increased osmolality of ionic contrast agents can result in osmotic hypervolemia and worsening congestive heart failure.

An emergency kit consisting of endotracheal tubes, Ambu bag, and emergency drugs including antihistamines, steroids, and IV fluids should be in the room when imaging exams requiring administration of ionic or nonionic contrast agents are performed. It is also recommended to have oxygen available and an intravenous catheter in place just in case an emergency arises.

Most of the contrast agents available on the market are intended for human use, but some are specifically approved by the U.S. Food and Drug Administration (FDA) for veterinary use. Many of the other products are used in veterinary medicine, though not specifically approved to do so. Never use out-of-date contrast media. Follow directions on the box insert to provide proper storage. Discard out-of-date contrast media just as you would any other out-of-date pharmaceutical.

Barium Sulfate

Barium sulfate, which is a water-insoluble salt of the metallic element barium, is the contrast medium used in examinations of the digestive tract if no perforation is suspected. It comes packaged as a powder or a liquid. A weight to volume measurement is generally the easiest way to mix barium to the desired density. Powdered barium cups have a line for several different densities, so adding water and mixing well is all that is necessary to prepare the barium sulfate for administration. 30–60% weight/volume barium sulfate suspension is typically used for stomach and small intestinal tract studies. 100% weight/volume is often used for large intestinal tract studies. Barium paste is often used for esophagrams, particularly if looking for a foreign body.

Oral ionic or nonionic contrast media should be used if a perforation is suspected in the GI tract. Oral ionic contrast media agents Gastrografin and MD-Gastroview and nonionic contrast media agent Omnipaque 180, 240, and 300 can be used orally or rectally. Omnipaque is currently the only nonionic low osmolar contrast media available with an oral indication in the United States for humans. It is water soluble, relatively nonabsorbable, and of low viscosity, which allows even coverage. It is also easily titrated to create the required density.

Special Imaging Procedures

Special Procedure—Esophagram (Static)

An esophagram is most useful to evaluate for esophageal motility, strictures, foreign bodies, perforations, or diverticuli.[5,10,14]

Contrast Agent: 45–85% barium sulfate suspension;[5,14] 60% weight/volume barium sulfate suspension is generally used.
Barium paste/esophageal cream.

Dosage: Canine: 15–30 ml, depending upon patient size.
Feline: 5–7 ml.[14]
Ferret: 3–4 ml w/curved tip dosing syringe.[14]

Precautions: Barium paste/esophageal cream should be used if foreign body is suspected. Ionic or nonionic contrast should be used if esophageal perforation is suspected. If oral ionic contrast media (Gastrografin or MD-Gastroview) is aspirated, pulmonary edema can result.[15] Oral nonionic contrast agent is safer and less toxic. Omnipaque 180, 240, or 300 (iohexol) can be used orally if diluted. Ionic or nonionic contrast media should be diluted 50:50 with water.[14]

Supplies: Canned and/or dry food in bowl mixed with liquid barium sulfate; canned food should be chunky in consistency.

Patient Prep: None.

General Procedural Instructions:

1. Take survey imaging views. Clinician preference. Thorax 2v and a lateral soft tissue neck are the more common views taken for imaging the esophagus.

2. Place patient in right lateral recumbent position.
3. Slowly administer liquid barium into lip fold.
4. Take lateral neck, lateral and VD or DV thorax immediately following the patient swallowing. Repeat views as needed to visualize the entire esophagus.
5. Place patient in right lateral recumbent position and administer barium paste/esophageal cream. Take lateral neck and lateral view of the thorax while the patient is swallowing.[5,10,14]
6. Feed the patient the barium/food mixture and immediately repeat radiographs. A 15- to 30-degree VD oblique view is recommended to assist in visualizing esophageal lesions.[14] Due to the possibility of aspiration, VD views may be contraindicated if the esophagus is dilated.[10]

Esophagram—Fluoroscopic/Dynamic

An esophagram is most useful to evaluate for esophageal motility, strictures, foreign bodies, perforations, or diverticuli. Fluoroscopic/dynamic imaging of the esophagus is most helpful in evaluating cricopharyngeal and esophageal function[5,10,14] (Figs. 16.1 and 16.2).

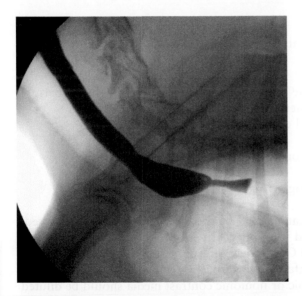

Figure 16.1. Fluoro esophagram with liquid barium.

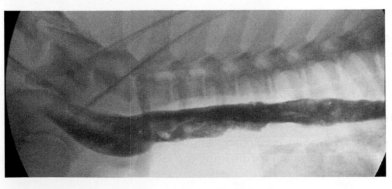

Figure 16.2. Fluoro esophagram with food mixture.

Contrast Agent: 45–85% barium sulfate suspension;[5,14] 60% weight/volume barium sulfate suspension is generally used.
Barium paste/esophageal cream.

Dosage: Canine: 15–30 mls, depending upon patient size.
Feline: 5–7 mls.[14]
Ferret: 3–4 mls w/curved tip dosing syringe.[14]

Precautions: Barium paste/esophageal cream should be used if foreign body is suspected. Ionic or nonionic contrast should be used if esophageal perforation is suspected. If oral ionic contrast media (Gastrografin or MD-Gastroview) is aspirated, pulmonary edema can result.[15] An oral nonionic contrast agent is safer and less toxic than Gastrografin or MD-Gastroview. Omnipaque 180 and 240 (iohexol) can be used orally if diluted. Ionic or nonionic contrast media should be diluted 50:50 with water.[14]

Supplies: Canned and/or dry food in bowl mixed with liquid barium sulfate; canned food should be chunky in consistency.

Patient Prep: None.

General Procedural Instructions:

1. Take survey imaging views. Clinician preference. Thorax 2v ± a lateral soft tissue neck are the more common views taken for evaluation of the esophagus.
2. Place patient in right lateral recumbent position.
3. Slowly administer liquid barium into lip fold.
4. Fluoroscopically monitor and record the administration of liquid barium, ± barium paste, ± barium mixed with food. It may take numerous swallows to evaluate esophageal motility and lower esophageal sphincter function.[14]

Special Procedure—Upper GI

An upper gastrointestinal study (**UGI**) is used to evaluate GI transit time, intestinal obstruction or masses, or possible foreign bodies. Normal gastric emptying time is 30–120 minutes. The normal small intestinal transit time is 30–120 minutes and emptying time is 180–300 minutes (Figs. 16.3 and 16.4).

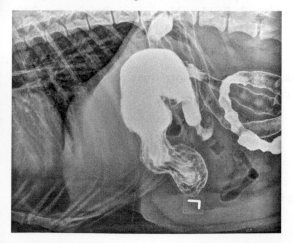

Figure 16.3.   UGI lateral view.

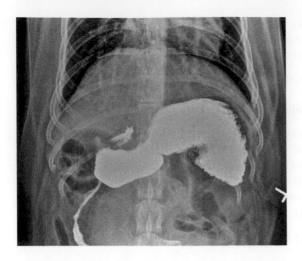

Figure 16.4.   UGI VD view.

Contrast Agent: 30%(feline)–60%(canine) barium sulphate.
Ionic or nonionic contrast media—diluted.

Dosage:

Barium Sulphate:

Canine: <20 kg: 8–12 ml/kg; >20 kg: 5–7 ml/kg.
Feline: 12–20 ml/kg.

Ionic or Nonionic Contrast Media:

Canine: ionic—Gastrografin or MD-Gastroview 3–5 ml/kg. Nonionic—Omnipaque 240(iohexol) 700–875 mgI/kg, diluted w/water for whole volume of 10 ml/kg.[14] 10 ml/kg 1:2 dilution.[5]

Feline: ionic—Gastrografin or MD-Gastroview 3–5 ml/kg. Nonionic—Omnipaque 240 (iohexol) 600–800 mgI/kg, diluted w/water for whole volume of 10 ml/kg.[14] 10 ml/kg 1:2 dilution.[5]

Precautions: Barium sulfate is contraindicated if a gastrointestinal perforation is suspected. An ionic or preferably a nonionic contrast media should be used.

Supplies:

Orogastric tube.
60 ml catheter tip syringes.

Patient Prep: Withhold food 12–24 hours; withhold water for 1–2 hours; enema, if necessary, 2–4 hours prior to study.

General Procedural Instructions:

1. Take VD and left lateral abdominal survey imaging views.
2. Slowly administer liquid barium orally or via orogastric tube.
3. Take right lateral, left lateral, DV, and VD views at 0 minutes.
4. Take right lateral and VD views at 15, 30, and 60 minutes after administering contrast media.
5. Continue taking images every 30 minutes until barium reaches the colon.[5,10,14]

Special Procedure—Gastrogram

A gastrogram is used to evaluate mucosal abnormalities of the stomach and rate of gastric emptying. Double contrast gastrography further evaluates the stomach wall for ulcers, masses, or foreign bodies. Negative contrast gastrography is used to evaluate the stomach walls and contents. If a GI perforation is suspected, do not use barium. Iodinated contrast (240–300 mgI/ml) should be diluted 50:50 with water (Fig. 16.5).

Contrast Agent:

Barium sulfate 30–60% weight/volume suspension for regular gastrogram.[5,10,14]
High-density barium of 100% weight/volume preferred for double contrast study, though not mandatory.[14]

Dosage:

Positive Contrast Gastrogram:

Canine/feline: barium sulfate 30% weight/volume 4–8 ml/kg.

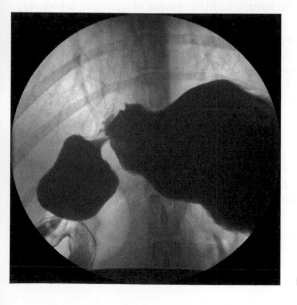

Figure 16.5.   Gastrogram fluoro image.

Double Contrast Gastrogram:

Canine: barium sulfate 100% weight/volume.
       <8 kg: 3.0 ml/kg; 8–40 kg: 2.0 ml/kg; >40 kg: 1.5 ml/kg.
Feline: 6 ml/kg using barium sulfate 100% weight/volume.
Ferret: 8–15 ml/kg via curved-tip dosing syringe using barium sulfate 30–60% weight/volume; 45 ml/kg air via orogastric tube 35 minutes post-contrast administration.[14]

Negative Contrast Gastrogram:

Canine/feline: 5–8 ml/kg of air; or carbonated soda (Mountain Dew or 7-Up); or effervescent granules or tablet.

Precautions: If perforation is suspected, do not use barium sulfate. If the stomach contains food, postpone the study.

Supplies:

Orogastric tube.
60 ml catheter tip syringes.
Curved-tip dosing syringe—ferret.
Air or carbon dioxide.

Patient Prep: Canine/feline: fast for 12 hours; patient should have water.
             Ferret: fast for 4 hours; patient should have water.

General Procedural Instructions:

1. Take VD and left lateral abdominal survey imaging views.
2. Administer liquid barium via orogastric tube.
3. Administer 20 ml/kg of air to distend the stomach. Effervescent granules or tablet may be used instead of air.
4. Remove tube and rotate patient 360 degrees along the long axis multiple times to coat the stomach.
5. Take DV, VD, right lateral, and left lateral views. If barium coating is inadequate, add an additional 1 ml/kg of barium.
6. Air should be removed via tube when the study is complete.

Special Instructions for Ferret:

1. Survey views should be VD and right lateral abdominal views.
2. Administer 8–15 ml/kg of barium via curved-tip dosing syringe.
3. Take right lateral and VD views of the abdomen at 0, 15, 30, and every 30 minutes until the barium reaches the colon.
4. Administer 45 ml/kg of air via the orogastric tube 35 minutes post-barium.
5. Take right and left lateral, DV, and VD views of the abdomen following air administration.[14]

Special Procedure—Lower GI—Barium Enema

Lower gastrointestinal studies are used to examine the colon for intussusceptions, strictures, or masses. The patient should be anesthetized for this study. Barium enemas can either be done as a positive contrast or double contrast imaging exam. Double contrast studies will further examine the bowel mucosa and wall thickness or identify strictures and masses (Figs. 16.6 and 16.7).

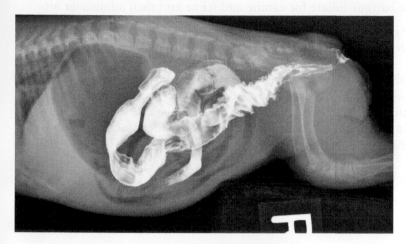

Figure 16.6. Lower GI lateral view.

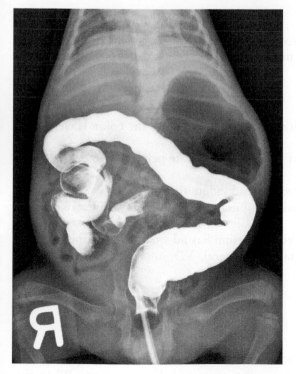

Figure 16.7.   Lower GI VD view.

Contrast Agent:

Canine/feline: 20–30% weight/volume barium sulfate or iodinated contrast.

Dosage:

Positive Barium Enema: Canine: 10–30 ml/kg rectally.
                          Feline: 7–11 ml/kg rectally.

Double Contrast Barium Enema: If no positive BE performed, administer 4–6 ml/kg of 20–25% weight/volume barium sulfate for canine and feline and then administer air.

Canine: 11 ml/kg of air is administered rectally.
Feline: 7–11 ml/kg of air is administered rectally.

Precautions: An air embolism can happen during any imaging exam using negative contrast. If the patient is suspected to have a portosystemic shunt, place the patient in a left lateral recumbent position to limit the chance of an air embolism. If an air embolism is seen, the patient should remain in a left lateral recumbent position for 60 minutes and immediate medical care should be initiated.[14]

Supplies:

Foley balloon-tip catheter.
60 ml syringes.
Exam gloves.
Lubricant.
Hemostat.

Patient Prep: Canine/feline: fast patient for 24 hours. Patient should be given water to keep well hydrated. If fecal material still in bowel when survey images are taken, give a warm-water enema.

General Procedural Instructions:

1. Take VD and right lateral survey abdominal images to ensure the colon is clean.
2. Anesthetize patient.
3. Place patient in right lateral recumbent position and elevate pelvis 10–15 degrees with a foam wedge.
4. Insert lubricated Foley catheter into rectum and inflate the bulb.
5. Place the syringe above the patient and, using gravity, administer barium.
6. Clamp tube.
7. Take right lateral abdominal view to verify barium has adequately filled the colon. If not, administer more barium. If so, take left lateral, VD, and oblique views of the abdomen.

Special Procedure—Excretory Urogram

The excretory urogram is also called an intravenous urogram or intravenous pyelogram. The study consists of two main phases, the nephrogram and the pyelogram. When the contrast agent is first injected, it should uniformly opacify the renal parenchyma within seconds as it is distributed in the renal vasculature. This is called the nephrogram phase. The contrast agent is then filtered into the renal collecting system with the urine and the renal pelvis and diverticula are opacified. This is called the pyelogram phase. The contrast agent then delineates the ureters and bladder, as it is excreted from the kidneys. If looking for ectopic ureters, no abdominal compression should be used during this study to allow a negative contrast cystogram to be performed post-excretory urogram. The excretory urogram will not provide quantitative data regarding renal function. If the patient's BUN or creatinine are highly elevated, the maximum dose of contrast media should be given as quickly as possible and images taken immediately post-injection (Figs. 16.8 and 16.9).

Contrast Agent: Ionic contrast agents: Conray, Conray 400, or Renografin 60.
Nonionic contrast agents: Ultravist 370, Isovue 370, Optiray 350, Omnipaque 240, or Visipaque 320.

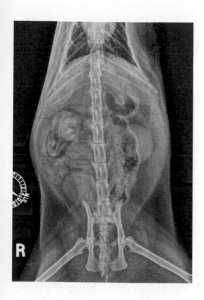

Figure 16.8.   IVU VD view.

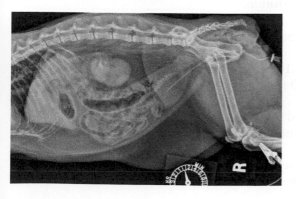

Figure 16.9.   IVU lateral view.

Dosage: Canine, feline, rabbit, and ferret: 880 mgI/kg (3 ml/kg).[5,14,10,15] One reference states the feline dose of 1 ml/kg is sufficient.[15]

Precautions: The study should not be performed on a dehydrated patient or one where renal function is seriously compromised. The intravenous catheter used for the injection should remain in place for at least 20 minutes post-contrast injection due to the incidence of adverse reactions. Vomiting is a frequent side effect of post-contrast injection. Caution should be used if planning to use a compression band for the pyelogram phase. Two references suggest using the compression band or abdominal pressure wrap to enhance the pyelogram phase, another reference stated compression is not recommended because it could cause worsen renal function temporarily, and a fourth reference does not mention using the compression band but also states a temporary decrease in renal function can occur post-excretory urography.[5,10,14,15]

Supplies:

Intravenous catheter w/injection cap.
Syringe w/needle.
Emergency drug kit.
Oxygen.

Patient Prep: Canine/feline: the patient should be fasted 24 hours prior to the study but can have water. A cleansing enema should be given at least 2 hours prior to the study. The patient should be assessed for dehydration; proceed only if well hydrated. An intravenous catheter should be placed just prior to study for contrast injection. The patient may require sedation if uncooperative.

Rabbit, guinea pig, ferret: a warm-water enema should be given after taking VD and right lateral survey images if fecal material in the colon. Recheck the colon in 1 hour.[14] The patient should be assessed for dehydration; proceed only if well hydrated. An intravenous catheter should be placed just prior to study for contrast injection. The patient may require sedation if uncooperative.

General Procedural Instructions:

1. Take VD and right lateral abdominal views to check colon for fecal material. If necessary, give another warm-water enema and recheck the colon in an hour. If clean, proceed.
2. Place the patient in a VD recumbent position.
3. Inject contrast media as a rapid bolus.
4. Take VD and right lateral views immediately post-injection. Oblique views may be taken 3–5 minutes post-injection.
5. Take VD and right lateral views at 5, 10 or 15, 20, and 30 minutes. Additional views may need to be taken at 45, 60, or 90 minutes if there is a delay in contrast enhancement of the renal system.
6. If using a compression band is desired due to poor filling of the renal pelvis, place it after the 5-minute views are taken and remove it just before taking the 10- or 15-minute views.
7. To help visualize ectopic ureters, a negative contrast cystogram can be done if no compression band was used during the study.

Special Procedure—Cystography

Cystography is performed to evaluate the urinary bladder using positive contrast, negative contrast, or a combination of both. Positive contrast cystography is used to visualize bladder position and the integrity of the bladder wall. A double contrast cystogram is best to provide mucosal detail and to visualize calculi and wall masses.[16] Negative contrast or pneumocystography is not often used due to the possibility of developing an air embolism, and it provides limited information. (Figs. 16.10 through 16.13).

Positive Contrast Cystography

Contrast Agent: Water-soluble ionic or nonionic contrast agents.

Dosage: Dilute contrast to 25% (1 part contrast to 3 parts sterile water or saline).[15,16]

Canine: 5–10 ml/kg.
Feline: 2–5 ml/kg.

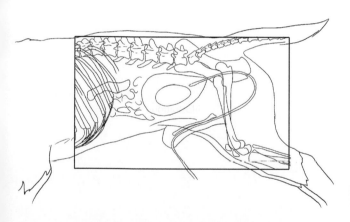

Figure 16.10.   Cystogram lateral illustration.

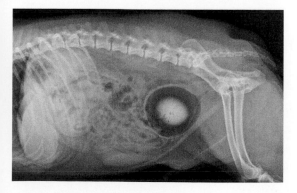

Figure 16.11.   Cystogram lateral view.

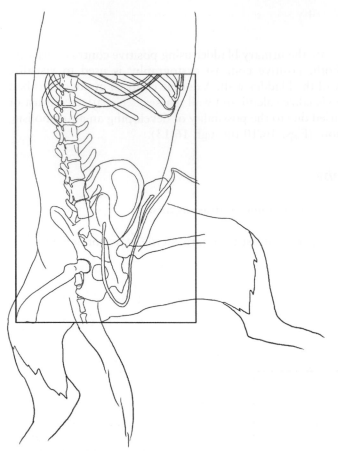

Figure 16.12. Cystogram oblique view illustration.

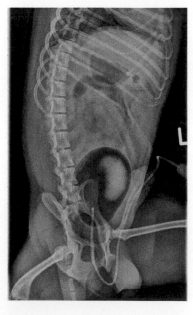

Figure 16.13. Cystogram oblique view.

Precautions: Palpate the bladder while administering the contrast agent to prevent rupture or overdistention of the bladder.

Supplies:

Sterile red rubber or polypropylene catheter, 3 1/2–5 French.
Sterile Christmas tree adapter.
3-way stopcock.
Syringes.
Sterile lubricant.
Germicidal soap and water prep.
Gauze.
2% lidocaine.
Sterile gloves.
Otoscope speculum.

Patient Prep: Patient should be fasted 12–24 hours and have cleansing enema(s) at least 4 hours prior to exam. Abdominal images should be taken prior to sedating or anesthetizing the patient to see if there is still fecal material over the bladder area. If so, a warm-water enema should be given and a second set of images should be taken in an hour to see if the colon is clean. The patient should be sedated or anesthetized for this procedure.

General Procedural Instructions:

1. Take right lateral and VD survey views of the abdomen.
2. The external area surrounding the urethra should be cleaned with a germicidal soap solution.
3. Using the sterile lubricant, aseptically catheterize and empty as much urine as possible from the bladder. It may be necessary to flush out any seen blood clots with sterile saline.
4. Administer 3–5 ml of 2% lidocaine into the bladder to reduce bladder straining due to distention for canine patients. 2–3 ml of 2% lidocaine should be used for feline patients.
5. The bladder should be held as the 25% diluted contrast agent is slowly administered to prevent overdistention.
6. Take right lateral, VD, and oblique views of the bladder. More contrast may have to be administered if there is leakage of contrast between views.
7. If following the positive cystogram with a double contrast cystogram, remove as much contrast agent as possible.
8. Turn patient onto the left side and re-inflate the bladder while palpating to prevent overdistention. An initial 5 ml/kg dosage is typical for canine patients and 2–3 ml/kg for feline patients.
9. Take lateral, VD, and oblique views of the bladder. More contrast may have to be administered if there is leakage of contrast between views.

Double Contrast Cystography

Contrast Agent: Air or soluble gas such as carbon dioxide.
                     Water-soluble ionic or nonionic contrast agents.

Dosage:

Air or Soluble Gas: 50–300 ml for larger dogs; 35 ml for small dogs and cats.

Ionic or Nonionic Contrast: Dilute contrast to 25% (1 part contrast to 3 parts sterile water or saline).[15,16]
1–2 ml for small dogs and cats.
2–10 ml for larger dogs.

Precautions: Palpate the bladder while administering the gas to prevent rupture or over-distention of the bladder. Place the patient in a left lateral recumbent position to administer gas to reduce the risk of an air embolism.[14]

Supplies:

Sterile red rubber or polypropylene catheter, 3 1/2–5 French.
Sterile Christmas tree adapter.
3-way stopcock.
Syringes.
Sterile lubricant.
Skin prep solution.
Gauze.
2% lidocaine.
Sterile gloves.
Otoscope speculum.

Patient Prep: Patient should be fasted 12–24 hours and have cleansing enema(s) at least 4 hours prior to exam. Abdominal images should be taken prior to sedating or anesthetizing the patient to see if there is still fecal material over the bladder area. If so, a warm-water enema should be given and a second set of images should be taken in an hour to see if the colon is clean. The patient should be sedated or anesthetized for this procedure.

General Procedural Instructions:

1. Take right lateral and VD survey views of the abdomen.
2. The external area surrounding the urethra should be cleaned with a germicidal soap solution.
3. Using the sterile lubricant, aseptically catheterize and empty as much urine as possible from the bladder. It may be necessary to flush out any seen blood clots with sterile saline.
4. Administer 3–5 ml of 2% lidocaine into the bladder to reduce bladder straining due to distention for canine patients. 2–3 ml of 2% lidocaine should be used for feline patients.
5. Place the patient in left lateral recumbent position to administer contrast agents.[14]
6. The bladder should be held as the air or soluble gas is slowly administered to prevent overdistention.
7. Slowly administer the ionic or nonionic contrast dosage and roll the patient 360 degrees to coat the mucosa with contrast.

8. Take left lateral, VD, and oblique views of the bladder. More contrast may have to be administered if there is leakage of contrast between views.

Pneumocystography

Air or soluble gas such as carbon dioxide.

Dosage: *Air or Soluble Gas:* 50–300 ml for larger dogs; 35 ml for small dogs and cats.

Precautions: Palpate the bladder while administering the gas to prevent rupture or over-distention of the bladder. Place the patient in a left lateral recumbent position to administer gas to reduce the risk of an air embolism.[14]

Supplies:

Sterile red rubber or polypropylene catheter, 3 1/2–5 French.
Sterile Christmas tree adapter.
3-way stopcock.
Syringes.
Sterile lubricant.
Germicidal soap and water prep.
Gauze.
2% lidocaine.
Sterile gloves.
Otoscope speculum.

Patient Prep: Patient should be fasted 12–24 hours and have cleansing enema(s) at least 4 hours prior to exam. Abdominal images should be taken prior to sedating or anesthetizing the patient to see if there is still fecal material over the bladder area. If so, a warm-water enema should be given and a second set of images should be taken in an hour to see if the colon is clean. The patient should be sedated or anesthetized for this procedure.

General Procedural Instructions:

1. Take right lateral and VD survey views of the abdomen.
2. The external area surrounding the urethra should be cleaned with a germicidal soap solution.
3. Using the sterile lubricant, aseptically catheterize and empty as much urine as possible from the bladder. It may be necessary to flush out any seen blood clots with sterile saline.
4. Administer 3–5 ml of 2% lidocaine into the bladder to reduce bladder straining due to distention for canine patients. 2–3 ml of 2% lidocaine should be used for feline patients.
5. Place the patient in left lateral recumbent position to administer air or soluble gas.[14]
6. The bladder should be held as the air or soluble gas is slowly administered to prevent overdistention.
7. Take left lateral, VD, and oblique views of the bladder. More contrast may have to be administered if there is leakage of gas between views.

CHAPTER 16

Special Procedure—Urethrography

Urethrography is performed to opacify the urethra to look for strictures, tears, and blockages due to calculi or masses. It can be performed as a supplemental study to cystography before or after the cystogram.

Visualizing the urethra, using ionic or nonionic contrast agents, can be done by retrograde or antegrade filling of the urethra. The antegrade or voiding cystourethrogram is performed post-positive contrast cystography. A radiolucent paddle is placed over the bladder to apply moderate pressure and a lateral view is taken when urine is seen at the urethral orifice. Air or soluble gas is rarely used for this study (Figs. 16.14 and 16.15).

Contrast Agent: Ionic or nonionic contrast agent: undiluted.

Dosage:

Ionic or Nonionic Contrast: Feline: 5 ml.
Small canine: 10 ml.

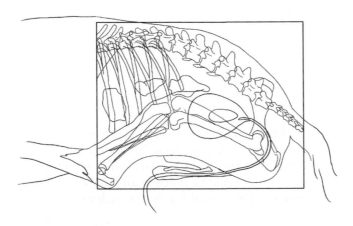

Figure 16.14.   Cystourethrogram flexed-leg illustration.

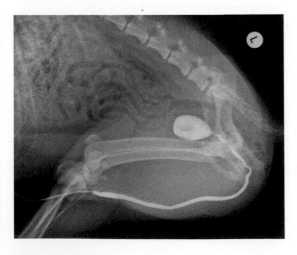

Figure 16.15.   Cystourethrogram flexed-leg view.

Medium canine: 20 ml.
Large canine: 30 ml.

Precautions: Excessive pressure should not be used for a voiding study, and it is contra-indicated to perform a voiding study if the bladder is severely diseased due to the increased likelihood of rupturing the bladder. Avoid producing air bubbles that may be mistaken for calculi when administered by prefilling the Foley catheter.

Supplies:

2% lidocaine.
Sterile lubricant.
3-way stopcock.
Syringes.
Skin prep solution.
Gauze.
Foley or Swan-Ganz balloon tip catheter.
Syringes.
Sterile gloves.
Otoscope speculum.

Patient Prep: Patient should be fasted 12–24 hours and have cleansing enema(s) at least 4 hours prior to exam. Abdominal images should be taken prior to sedating or anesthetizing the patient to see if there is still fecal material in the distal colon and rectum. The patient should be sedated for this exam.

General Procedural Instructions:

1. Take right lateral (regular and flexed-leg) and VD survey views of the abdomen.
2. The external area surrounding the urethra should be cleaned with a germicidal soap solution.
3. Prefill the Foley catheter with contrast prior to dipping the tip in a sterile lubricant and aseptically placing it just beyond the urethral papilla in females or within the penile urethra in males. This will prevent the injection of air bubbles.
4. Inject 2 ml of 2% lidocaine into the urethra.
5. Position the patient for the flexed lateral view.
6. Inject 50% of the contrast dosage and make the exposure near the end of the injection.
7. Inject contrast again, taking another flexed-leg lateral to evaluate if previous filling defects are still present.
8. Proceed in taking regular right lateral, VD, and/or oblique views of the bladder, as necessary, administering more contrast for each view.

Special Procedure—Vaginography

A vaginogram or retrograde vaginourethrogram is a contrast study performed to examine the vagina, cervix, and urethra to look for ectopic ureters, vaginal strictures or masses, and vaginal or urethral tears (Figs. 16.16 through 16.18).

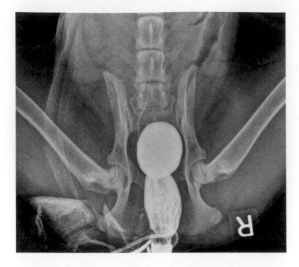

Figure 16.16.   Vaginogram VD view.

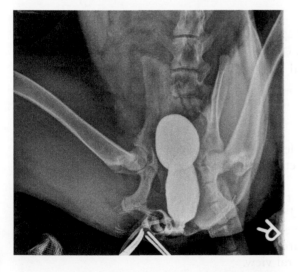

Figure 16.17.   Vaginogram oblique view.

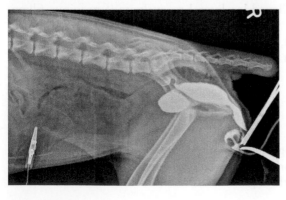

Figure 16.18.   Vaginogram lateral view.

Contrast Agent: Ionic or nonionic contrast agent: undiluted.

Dosage:

Ionic or Nonionic Contrast:

Feline: 5 ml.
Small canine: 10 ml.
Medium canine: 20 ml.
Large canine: 30 ml.

Precautions: Avoid producing air bubbles that may be mistaken for calculi when administered by prefilling the Foley catheter.

Supplies:

Sterile lubricant.
Syringes.
Germicidal soap and water prep.
Gauze.
Foley or Swan-Ganz balloon tip catheter.
Sterile gloves.

Patient Prep: Patient should be fasted 12–24 hours and have cleansing enema(s) at least 4 hours prior to exam. Abdominal images should be taken prior to sedating or anesthetizing the patient to see if there is still fecal material in the distal colon and rectum. The patient should be anesthetized for this procedure.

General Procedural Instructions:

1. Take right lateral and VD survey views of the abdomen.
2. The external area surrounding the urethra should be cleaned with a germicidal soap solution.
3. Aseptically catheterize the bladder to remove as much urine as possible and then remove catheter.[14]
4. Prefill the Foley catheter with contrast prior to placing it in the vulva. Inflate the cuff just inside the vestibule.
5. Inject the undiluted contrast dose to adequately fill the vagina.
6. Proceed in taking a right lateral view of the caudal abdomen near the end of the injection. Take VD and/or oblique views, as necessary.[10,14,15,16]

Special Procedure—Myelography

Myelography is a contrast study used to examine the spinal cord by injecting nonionic contrast media into the subarachnoid space. This study is used to identify sites of cord compression due to spinal cord swelling, protruding disk material, vertebral abnormality, or mass. A myelogram should only be performed by an experienced clinician intending to take the patient to surgery if a surgical lesion is identified.

CHAPTER 16

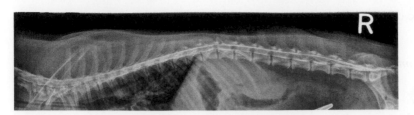

Figure 16.19.   Myelogram
TL lateral view.

The contrast agent is injected either at a cisternal or lumbar site. For injections at the cisternal site, which is located between the external occipital protuberance and the arch of C1, the patient is in a lateral recumbent position with the head hyperflexed. For injections at the lumbar site, which is located between L5 and 6, the patient is placed in either a sternal recumbent position or a lateral recumbent position with the lumbar spine flexed with the hind legs extended cranially to open the interarcuate space. The lumbar site is preferred over the cisternal site (Figs. 16.19 through 16.21).

Contrast Agent: Iohexol (Omnipaque 240 mgI/ml) or iopamidol (Isovue 200 mgI/ml). **Only nonionic iodinated contrast agents with an iodine concentration of 200–300 mgI/kg** and approved for intrathecal use.

Dosage: Canine and feline: cisternal injection—cervical spine, 0.3 ml/kg; TL spine, 0.45 ml/ kg. Lumbar injection—cervical spine, 0.45 ml/kg; TL spine, 0.3 ml/kg.

Precautions: Procedure should only be performed by an experience clinician. Seizures may occasionally occur during recovery, particularly if the contrast agent entered the skull. Make sure nonionic contrast agent chosen is approved for intrathecal use.

Supplies:

Spinal needle 20–22 g.
Clippers.
Surgical scrub.
Sterile gloves.
Venotube for CSF collection.

Patient Prep: Patient must be anesthetized. Either a cisternal or lumbar injection site should be clipped and aseptically prepared. For a cisternal injection, the area between the cranial edge of the ears to a point halfway down the neck should be clipped and aseptically prepped. For a lumbar injection, the dorsal midline from the midlumbar area to the caudal end of the sacrum should be clipped and aseptically prepped.

General Procedural Instructions:

1. Anesthetize the patient.
2. Take VD and right lateral survey views of the spine.
3. Clip and aseptically prep the injection site.
4. Clinician will aseptically place the spinal needle in the subarachnoid space and may collect CSF for cytology analysis.
5. If performing a static study, the clinician will inject 0.2–0.5 ml of the contrast agent to confirm proper placement of the needle. A lateral view of the spine centered at the

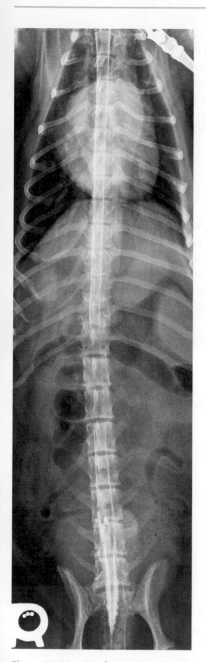

Figure 16.20.   Myelogram TL VD view.

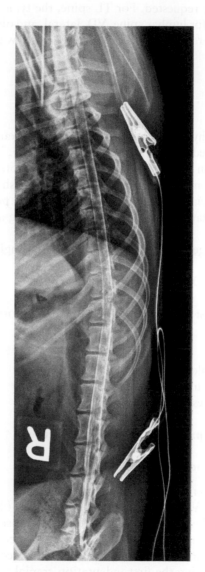

Figure 16.21.   Myelogram TL oblique view.

injection site will confirm the needle is in the subarachnoid space. If not, the needle will be repositioned by the clinician and another image is taken to confirm the needle is properly placed. The contrast agent is injected slowly, taking approximately 1 minute to complete the injection.[15,16] The patient is not to be moved during injection and while the spinal needle is still placed.

6. A lateral view is taken at the end of the injection to confirm adequate filling of the subarachnoid space. After the needle has been removed, it may be necessary to tilt the body to facilitate better filling of the subarachnoid space at a particular site.

7. For cervical spine, VD, lateral, oblique, flexion, extension, and traction, lateral views may be requested. For TL spine, the typical views taken are VD, lateral, and oblique views; for lumbar spine, VD, lateral, and oblique views. If a spinal fracture is suspected, the lateral view and horizontal beam view to attain a VD projection may be requested.

Special Procedure—Myelography—Avian[14,17,18]

Myelography is a contrast study used to examine the spinal cord by injecting nonionic contrast media into the subarachnoid space. This study is used to identify sites of cord compression due to spinal cord swelling, protruding disk material, vertebral abnormality, or mass. A myelogram on an avian patient should only be performed by a vastly experienced clinician. Myelography should not be performed on ducks, geese, or swans due to the bone plates overlapping, thereby limiting access to the injection site.[14]

Contrast Agent: Iohexol (Omnipaque 240 mgI/ml) should be used for this procedure.

Dosage: 190–280 mgI/kg.[14]

Precautions: Procedure should only be performed by a vastly experienced clinician.

Supplies:

Spinal needle 25 gauge, 1.5 inch.
Surgical scrub.
Sterile gloves.

Patient Prep: Patient must be anesthetized.

General Procedural Instructions:

1. Anesthetize the patient.
2. Take DV and right lateral survey views of the spine.
3. Place the patient in ventral recumbent position and restrain the patient in this position.
4. Pluck and aseptically prep the 3 cm injection site located over the junction between the notarium and the synsacrum. The injection site is found by palpating the ilial crests and finding the first indentation cranial to the synsacrum.
5. Clinician will aseptically place the spinal needle in indentation. CSF within the spinal needle should be confirmed prior to injection.
6. The clinician will inject a small amount of contrast agent and request a DV view of the injection site be taken to confirm proper placement of the needle. The contrast agent is injected slowly, and the bird is not to be moved during injection while the spinal needle is still in place. Additional DV views may be requested during the process.
7. The spinal needle is removed once the injection is complete.
8. Take a DV and lateral views of the spine post-injection.

Special Procedure—Myelography—Rabbit

Myelography is a contrast study used to examine the spinal cord by injecting nonionic contrast media into the subarachnoid space. This study is used to identify sites of cord compression due to spinal cord swelling, protruding disk material, vertebral abnormality, or mass. A myelogram should only be performed on a rabbit by a vastly experienced clinician.

The contrast agent is injected either at a cisternal or lumbar site. For injections at the cisternal site, which is located between the external occipital protuberance and the arch of C1, the patient is in a lateral recumbent position with the head hyperflexed. For rabbits, injections at the lumbar site, which is located between L5 and 6, is preferred.

Contrast Agent: Iohexol (Omnipaque 240 mgI/ml) or iopamidol (Isovue 200 mgI/ml). **Only nonionic iodinated contrast agents with an iodine concentration of 200–300 mgI/kg and approved for intrathecal use.**

Dosage: 0.2 ml/kg.

Precautions: Procedure should only be performed on a rabbit by a vastly experienced clinician. Seizures may occasionally occur during recovery, particularly if the contrast agent entered the skull. Make sure nonionic contrast agent chosen is approved for intrathecal use.

Supplies:

Spinal needle 20–22 g.
Clippers.
Surgical scrub.
Sterile gloves.
Venotube for CSF collection.

Patient Prep: Patient must be anesthetized. The lumbar injection site should be clipped and aseptically prepared. For a lumbar injection, the dorsal midline from the midlumbar area to the caudal end of the sacrum should be clipped and aseptically prepped.

General Procedural Instructions:

1. Anesthetize the patient.
2. Take VD and right lateral survey views of the spine.
3. Clip and aseptically prep the injection site.
4. Clinician will aseptically place the spinal needle in the subarachnoid space and may collect CSF for cytology analysis.
5. If performing a static study, the clinician will inject 0.2–0.5 ml of the contrast agent to confirm proper placement of the needle. A lateral view of the spine centered at the injection site will confirm the needle is in the subarachnoid space. If not, the needle will be repositioned by the clinician and another image is taken to confirm the needle is properly placed. The contrast agent is injected slowly, taking approximately 1 minute to complete the injection.[15,16] The patient cannot be moved during injection and while the spinal needle is still placed.

6. A lateral view is taken at the end of the injection to confirm adequate filling of the subarachnoid space. After the needle has been removed, it may be necessary to tilt the body to facilitate better filling of the subarachnoid space at a particular site.
7. For cervical, TL, and lumbar spines, VD, lateral, and oblique views may be requested. If a spinal fracture is suspected, the lateral view and horizontal beam view to attain a VD projection may be requested.

Special Procedure—Fistulography

A fistula is deep sinuous passage or draining tract exiting at the skin's surface from an abscess or hollow organ. Sometimes a fistula will be a congenital pathway between two organs. Radiolucent foreign bodies or sequestra associated with osteomyelitis can frequently cause a fistula. To find the origin of the fistula, a contrast agent is injected into the tract to opacify the tract and find the source (Figs. 16.22 and 16.23).

Contrast Agent: Water-soluble ionic or nonionic iodinated contrast agent.

Dosage: Dependent upon size of tract.

Precautions: NA.

Supplies:

Syringes.
Foley catheter.

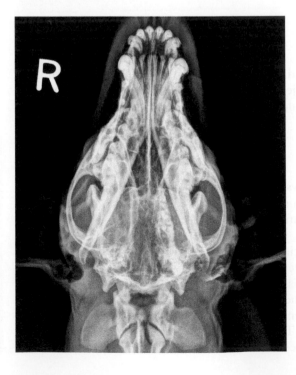

Figure 16.22.   Fistulogram DV view.

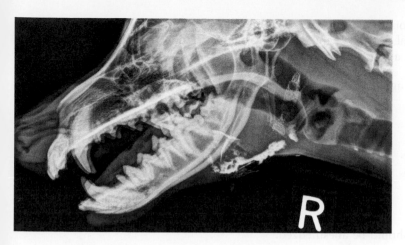

Figure 16.23.   Fistulogram lateral view.

Clippers.
Skin prep solution.
Metallic marker.

Patient Prep: Sedation is usually necessary. Clip the hair and debris from the opening of the draining tract and cleanse the site. Place a metallic marker, like a BB, at the opening of the tract.

General Procedural Instructions:

1. Take VD or craniocaudal and lateral views of the anatomic region to determine the size of the tract and cavity.
2. Insert a flexible balloon tip catheter, like a Foley, into the tract and advance it in as far as it will go. Inflate the balloon to help prevent leakage of the contrast agent.
3. Inject the tract with contrast agent volume to adequately fill the tract.
4. Immediately take post-contrast views to include a lateral and VD or craniocaudal views. After removing the catheter, repeat the views.
5. Air or soluble gas can be injected after the contrast if a double contrast exam is needed. The volume of air/gas will be the same as the iodinated contrast agent.

Special Procedure—Arthrography

Arthrography is a contrast study of a joint cavity using positive or negative contrast media to outline the joint capsule, to identify the articular surfaces, and to visualize free bodies within the joint. The shoulder and stifle joints are the most common joints studied. Arthrograms are not performed as frequently as in the past due to the availability of MRI and CT.

Contrast Agent: Diluted nonionic contrast.

Dosage: 1–4 ml of a nonionic contrast agent diluted to 140 mgI/ml for shoulder joint and 0.4 ml/kg of 100 mgI/ml for the bicipital groove. The nonionic contrast agent should be diluted 1 part contrast agent to 2 parts isotonic sterile saline.

Precautions: Contrast agent must be diluted to prevent damage to intracapsular ligaments or damaged cartilage.

Supplies:

22 gauge spinal needle.
Surgical scrub supplies.
Clippers.
Syringes.

Patient Prep: Patient should be anesthetized.

General Procedural Instructions:

Shoulder:

1. The patient is anesthetized.
2. Lateral and caudocranial survey images are taken of the shoulder.
3. The lateral aspect of the shoulder is aseptically prepared as the injection site.
4. The clinician will aseptically place the 22 gauge spinal needle in the joint at the point of interest. Withdrawing joint fluid or taking an image after injecting a small amount of contrast will confirm proper needle placement.
5. Remove the needle and manipulate the joint to uniformly fill the joint space with the contrast agent.
6. Take lateral, caudocranial, and oblique views of the joint.

Stifle:

1. The patient is anesthetized.
2. Lateral and caudocranial survey images are taken of the stifle.
3. Aseptically prepare the injection site.
4. The clinician will aseptically place the 20 or 22 gauge, 1 inch needle midway between the cranial point of the patella and the tibial tuberosity, just medial to the patellar ligament.
5. Withdrawing joint fluid or taking an image after injecting a small amount of contrast will confirm proper needle placement.
6. The clinician will inject 1.4–1.8 ml/joint of nonionic iodinated contrast media 280 mgI/ml over 10–20 seconds.[14,15]
7. The clinician will remove the needle and manipulate the joint to uniformly fill the joint space with the contrast agent.
8. Take lateral and caudocranial views of the joint within 5 minutes post-injection.[14,15,18]

References

1. Carter, Christi E., and Beth L. Veale. 2010. *Digital Radiography and PACS*. St. Louis: Mosby.
2. Bushong, Stewart C. 2001. *Radiologic Science for Technologists: Physics, Biology, and Protection*, 7th ed. St. Louis: Mosby.
3. Fauber, Terri L. 2009. *Radiographic Imaging & Exposure*, 3rd ed. St. Louis: Mosby.
4. Korner, Markus, Christof H. Weber, Stefan Wirth, Klaus-Jurgen Pfeifer, Maximilian Reiser, and Marcus Treitl. RSNA 2007. Advances in Digital Radiography; Physical Principles and System Overview. *RadioGraphics* 27:675–686.
5. Thrall, Donald E. 2007. *Textbook of Veterinary Diagnostic Radiology*, 5th ed. St. Louis: Saunders.
6. Puchalski, Sarah M. December 1, 2006. Exploring Your Digital Radiography Equipment Options. Veterinary Medicine Supplement. http://veterinarymedicine.dvm360.com.
7. Shiroma, Jonathan T. December 1, 2006. An Introduction to DICOM. Veterinary Medicine Supplement. http://veterinarymedicine.dvm360.com.
8. Wallack, Seth T. December 1, 2006. How to Store Digital Images and Comply with Medical Recordkeeping Standards. Veterinary Medicine Supplement. http://veterinary medicine.dvm360.com.
9. Cahoon, John B. 1974. *Formulating X-ray Techniques*, 8th ed. Durham, NC: Duke University Press.
10. Lavin, Lisa M. 2003. *Radiography in Veterinary Technology*, 3rd ed. St. Louis: Saunders.
11. Artifact image file courtesy of Dr. Jeryl Jones, DVM, PhD, DACVR; Professor of Veterinary Radiology; West Virginia University, Morgantown, WV.
12. Artifact image file courtesy of Mary H. Ayers, R.T. (R); Veterinary Teaching Hospital, Virginia-Maryland Regional College of Veterinary Medicine, Blacksburg, VA.
13. Jensen, Steven C., and Michael P. Peppers. 1998. *Pharmacology and Drug Administration for Imaging Technologists*. St. Louis: Mosby.
14. Wallack, Seth T. 2003. *The Handbook of Veterinary Contrast Radiography*. San Diego Veterinary Imaging, Inc.
15. Morgan, J.P., and Sam Silverman. 1987. *Techniques of Veterinary Radiography*, 4th ed. Ames: Iowa State University Press.
16. Owens, Jerry M., and Darryl N. Biery. 1999. *Radiographic Interpretation for the Small Animal Clinician*, 2nd ed. Philadelphia: Lippincott Williams & Wilkins.
17. Rubel, G.A., E. Isenbugel, and P. Wolvekamp. 1991. *Atlas of Diagnostic Radiology of Exotic Pets*. St. Louis: Saunders.

18. Harr, K.E., G.V. Kollias, V. Rendano, and A. DeLahunta. 1997. Myelographic Technique for Avian Species. *Veterinary Radiology and Ultrasound* 38(3):187–192.
19. Wright, Matt, and William J. Hornof. 2010. *Purchasing Digital Radiography without Getting Your Head Handed to You.* San Diego: Animal Insides Press.
20. Wright, Matt. 2010. *Digital Radiography for the Veterinary Technician.* San Diego: Animal Insides Press.
21. Wright, Matt. 2008. *Radiation Safety and Non-Manual Patient Restraint in Veterinary Radiography.* San Diego: Animal Insides Press.
22. "Edison Fears the Hidden Perils of the X-rays." August 3, 1903. New York World, Duke University Rare Book, Manuscript, and Special Collections Library, Durham, NC.
23. Hall, Eric J. 2000. *Radiobiology for the Radiologist,* 5th ed. Philadelphia: Lippincott Williams & Wilkins.

Webliography

www.animalinsides.com/learn/general-imaging. Evaluating the Improperly Exposed Radiograph.
www.offa.org/hd_procedures.html. Orthopedic Foundation for Animals.
www.PennHIP.org. PennHIP, the University of Pennsylvania, School of Veterinary Medicine.

Index

Printed and bound by CPI Group (UK) Ltd, Croydon, CR0 4YY

27/10/2024

14580243-0001